GUIDE TO NEUROLOGICAL ASSESSMENT

HOWARD S. BARROWS, M.D.

Professor of Medicine (Neurology)
McMaster University Medical Centre
Hamilton, Ontario, Canada

GUIDE TO NEUROLOGICAL ASSESSMENT

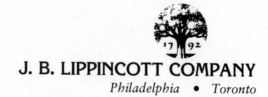

J. B. LIPPINCOTT COMPANY
Philadelphia • *Toronto*

3   4   5   6

Library of Congress Cataloging in Publication Data

Barrows, Howard S
    Guide to neurological assessment.

    Bibliography:
    Includes index.
    1. Neurologic examination. I. Title. [DNLM: 1. Neurologic examination.
WL141 B278g]
RC348.B325   616.8'04754   80-13273
ISBN 0-397-52093-X

The author and publisher have exerted every effort to ensure that drug selection
and dosage set forth in this text are in accord with current recommendations and
practice at the time of publication. However, in view of ongoing research,
changes in government regulations, and the constant flow of information relating
to drug therapy and drug reactions, the reader is urged to check the package in-
sert for each drug for any change in indications and dosage and for added warn-
ings and precautions. This is particularly important when the recommended agent
is a new or infrequently employed drug.

PREFACE

This book began fifteen years ago as a guide for clinical clerks on neurology, and has slowly evolved into its present form on the basis of continuing personal experience in teaching medical students and house staff. Their direct feedback has lead to many modifications to meet expressed needs.

The book was written to provide a reference that both served as a ready brief guide on how to perform the neurologic examination and, at the same time, provide enough basic information about the mechanisms involved in the examination to permit the student to synthesize the data he accumulates from the patient and to localize the responsible lesion.

I would like to give special thanks to Alison Barrows for all the illustrations on the examination of the patient, and to Paul Knowles for the wiring diagrams. I owe a great debt to Phyllis Barrows for her endless encouragement to get this book written in publishable form, for manuscript review, and for endless final typing.

CONTENTS

GUIDE TO
NEUROLOGICAL
ASSESSMENT

1

HISTORY TAKING AND THE NEUROLOGICAL EXAMINATION

HISTORY TAKING

There are many resources available on general techniques in history taking. However, in taking a neurological history, you, the examiner, should remember the following points:

1. The course of the patient's illness and the interrelated course of each symptom should be carefully documented (temporal profile). This profile can provide the important clues to etiology (Fig. 1-1). At best, the neurological examination can only indicate the location and extent of neural damage; it rarely gives any etiological clues.

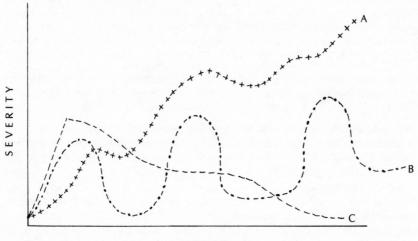

Fig. 1-1. Temporal profiles. *(A)* A relentlessly progressive course can suggest neoplastic or degenerative disease. *(B)* Recurrent attacks with increasing deficit between attacks can suggest demyelinating or vascular disease. *(C)* Sudden onset with progressive clearing (or worsening) is seen in infections and vascular disease.

2. Careful search for the earliest symptoms of neurological disease must always be made. Fluctuating, chronic, insidious diseases can be present for many years and produce only a few dramatic symptoms in the patient. This is usually because the patient has either adapted to the symptoms or forgotten when they first appeared. This search may require assiduous questioning and possibly questioning of the family or close contacts.
3. Stigmata of neurological disease in members of the family must be carefully sought. Again, this often necessitates inquiry of other members of the family. Considerable effort, time, and discomfort to the patient may be spared by the discovery that his condition is hereditary. Almost every symptom complex in neurology can be mimicked by a hereditary condition.
4. Direct questioning about all important neurological symptoms must be done before history taking is finished. For example, you must inquire about the symptoms listed below:

Important Neurological Symptoms

Headache
Dizziness
Seizure or seizure-like episodes, and transient involuntary changes in consciousness or behavior
Altered consciousness
Disordered mentation: personality change, memory loss, confusion
Weakness
Sensory phenomena or disordered sensations
Altered libido, sexual dysfunction, or menstrual irregularities
Sphincter disturbances
Disorders of sight and hearing (*e.g.,* scotoma, diplopia, tinnitus)
Disorders of olfaction
Difficulty in performance of daily motor activities
Difficulty in speech, swallowing, and chewing
Insomnia, drowsiness, and disorders of sleep
Tremors and involuntary movements

In his concern about his present difficulty, the patient may have forgotten other symptoms that could be important to understanding his neurological problem, or he might have felt they were too trivial to mention.

5. Never accept the patient's word for such symptoms as numbness or dizziness without carefully determining what the patient is actually experiencing. The connotation of many words for symptoms vary widely. However, the true nature of the symptom as a subjective experience can be crucial to your analysis. For example, "dizziness" can mean such widely divergent sensations as vertigo, syncope, unsteadiness, or confusion. The pathophysiological significance of each is markedly different. "Numbness" may mean loss of sensation, paresthesia, or weakness of a limb with no sensory phenomena.
6. Always be concerned about how you mentally "translate" the patient's symptoms into convenient medical jargon for your own thinking and your records. In doing this, you might alter the symptom's true significance. With each symptom, you should inquire about the following aspects of the patient's symptoms:

Onset
Exact nature or character of the symptom
Severity
Relationship to other events, time, meals, postural change
Location in body at onset, and change in pattern over time
Associated symptoms
What relieves; what aggravates
Temporal profile

The questioning style of each examiner is usually unique, in keeping with his personality and conversational style. However, two final points must be kept in mind when interviewing the patient:

7. Avoid suggesting responses to the patient by the way the question is phrased (*e.g.*, "Did your headache come on suddenly?"). It is better to approach such information obliquely: "How did your headache begin?" Offer the patient alternatives, such as, "Did your headaches begin gradually or rapidly?" Symptoms are often hard to describe, and if you ask, "Was the pain knife-like?," the patient may accept your definition rather than tell you with difficulty, but more accurately, how it really felt. Keep potential traps like these always in mind.

8. Do not finish your questioning until you can literally put yourself in the patient's place and experience his illness. You must have complete understanding of how the illness began, developed, and affected the patient. Question in any way necessary to fill gaps in understanding. If you have enough information to simulate the patient for another physician, you have understood his illness well.

THE NEUROLOGICAL EXAMINATION

Since the central nervous system is located behind bone, it cannot be visualized (except for the optic discs), palpated, percussed, or auscultated as can other tissues. Therefore, its intactness can be deduced only by functional testing. The major part of the neurological examination is a technique of stimulus-response from the simplest reflex to complex stimuli and responses requiring cortical integration. The examiner's success in the neurological examination depends on a thorough knowledge of the range of normal responses, and the use of a standardized basic technique with every patient. The basic neurological examination for a patient with no particular symptoms or findings (a screening routine) is suggested in chapter 10. As the student becomes more experienced, he will modify his examination to suit the problem the patient presents. He can then focus on the problem areas and screen for other neurological abnormalities. Success also depends on the examiner's ability to communicate his instructions to the patient clearly and simply. This requires constant thought and practice.

When the patient first enters the room, your examination begins. The patient's facial expression may indicate emotions, depression, hostility, or it may indicate one of the characteristic facies of myasthenia gravis, muscular dystrophy, hyperthyroidism, Cushing's syndrome, or bulbar paralysis. Body symmetry and the patient's ease in walking and sitting can give important early clues about neurological deficits, as does the strength and quality of the handshake (often the first clue to myotonia). The posture of the patient should be noted, as well as the manner in which the hands are held or used. This can be priceless information—don't miss it!

As you examine the patient, remember that such concepts as "sensory" and "motor" are arbitrary terms used as a taxonomic convenience to indicate whether the series of neural impulses or messages are going to the central nervous system from sensory receptors or whether the impulses are going from the central nervous system to influence muscle contraction. The nervous system is complex and integrated; deficits anywhere can affect motor performance.

The presentation in this book is organized by anatomical systems (*e.g.*, motor, reflexes, sensory, cranial nerves, mental functions) so that the student will understand how data from the neurological examination can identify underlying altered anatomy. The examiner should organize his neurological examination in a sequence and manner that appeals to him and do it consistently. If the patient has paralyzed legs, start with the legs. If the patient has back pain, start with the back. If the patient is confused or aphasic, start with mental status. Order is not as important as tailoring the examination to the patient's problem.

Chapter 13 describes how the clinician employs the scientific method to understand and resolve the patient's neurological problem, utilizing the techniques described in this book to obtain the data necessary for this reasoning process. This chapter also describes helpful strategies in facilitating this process with neurological patients. Within the next ten chapters there are discussions on the technique of the examination to help you analyze and synthesize the data you obtain from your examination of the patient. These discussions are in contrasting type.

2

THE MOTOR SYSTEM

INSPECTION OF THE STANDING PATIENT

The appearance of the entire body, and the manner in which the motor system maintains the antigravity posture, can give clues concerning the nature and extent of the patient's disability. The examiner should look for the following things when he inspects the standing, disrobed patient:

1. Postural abnormalities (*e.g.*, the flexed, stooped posture of the parkinsonian patient, and the lumbar lordosis and sagging shoulders of the patient with proximal muscle paralysis).
2. Musculoskeletal abnormalities (*e.g.*, scoliosis, lordosis, kyphosis, muscle or joint contractures, abnormal head posture, high arched feet, short neck, malformations of the cranium, gibbus, abnormal carrying angle, and saber shins).
3. Proportion and appearance of body parts (*e.g.*, contour of muscles, muscle atrophy, fat distribution, hair distribution, relative size of body parts, apparent age, primary and secondary sexual development).
4. Skin appearance (*e.g.*, nevi, rashes, tumors, birthmarks, café-au-lait spots, lipomata, cysts, tufts of hair, texture and color of the skin).
5. Abnormal muscle movements (*e.g.*, tics, choreic movements, tremors, fasciculations). Unless the entire musculature is visualized, the fleeting abnormal movements of chorea or fasciculations, especially on the trunk, could be missed.

INSPECTION OF GAIT

The patient's gait is a highly integrated motor performance. Subtle disorders in many different systems can express themselves in characteristic gait disturbances. The examiner should look for right-left symmetry, in the swing of the arms, the distance the feet are spread from the midline in walking (gait base), reciprocal arm motion in relation to leg movement, stability of the pelvis and shoulders during walking, thoracic stability in side-to-side movement, and placement of the heel followed by controlled placement of the toes on the floor. Be certain that the patient's arms are not inhibited by having to hold a gown closed or carry a handkerchief. The arms should be free at the sides.

Corticospinal system dysfunction producing hemiparesis can be manifested by audible foot dragging or toe scuffing due to early dorsiflexor weakness; reduced or lost reciprocal or associated arm swing (swing in the same direction of the arm opposite the leg); and circumduction movement of the leg. A hemiplegic limp or posture can be seen if the dysfunction is more marked.

Cerebellar system dysfunction can be indicated by a broad-based gait (normally feet are placed quite close to the midline in walking); irregular foot placement while walking (ataxia); and poor turning at the end of walking, usually requiring extra steps associated with instability or drifting to one or both sides (most people reverse their walking with a simple two-step turn). The patient often cannot keep the body's center of gravity within the area of foot support. Characteristically, the arms are held out from the sides during walking. Even when the arms are put out for balance, it may be performed in an incoordinated, clumsy manner. The body may show irregular oscillations of the trunk on standing (truncal ataxia). Such patients must be watched closely to prevent falls; often the examiner needs to offer some support. On standing, the normal subject displays an appropriate fine play of tendon movements over the dorsal aspect of the feet as cerebellar coordinated reflexes automatically maintain the erect stance. In patients with cerebellar disease, these movements may be inappropriate, delayed, or exaggerated with over-correction. With mild cerebellar dysfunction, this finding can be brought out by giving the standing patient a push. In unilateral cerebellar disease, positive findings are found on the side of the lesion. Sometimes the head may be inclined sideways to the side of the lesion. Truncal and gait ataxia without significant arm ataxia suggest midline (vermis) or anterior lobe involvement of the cerebellum.

A patient's gait can show signs of both corticospinal and cerebellar dysfunctions in diseases affecting both pathways in the spinal cord or brain stem, producing a "spastic-cerebellar gait." This combination may be hard to disentangle without other evidences of corticospinal or cerebellar dysfunction in the examination.

Extrapyramidal system dysfunction may show the characteristic signs of parkinsonism (e.g., a shuffling gait, "Marche à petits pas," retropulsion, propulsion, and loss of associated movements of the arms). Patients with these signs may also show akinesia, a poverty of spontaneous automatic movement, and a marked effort in initiating voluntary movements, even though there is no weakness. Other extrapyramidal signs on walking include dystonic postures with bizarre inversion of the foot, hyperflexion of the knee and hip, and tremors and hyperkinesias (see p. 12).

Muscle weakness in the distal lower extremities can be characterized by a "slapping gait" caused by weakness of the dorsiflexors of the foot. In walking, the dorsiflexors are unable to control the rapid descent of the toes after the heel has touched the ground. Patients with these signs may show poor ankle stability. When the dorsiflexors become ineffective, the feet hang down, and over-flexion of the knee is required to clear the toe from the ground with each step ("steppage gait"). Any limp can appear to be a gait of neurologic significance; shortness of the leg, joint or muscle pains, joint limitations, and foot deformity must be ruled out. Subsequent areas of examination can help sort out possible sources of gait difficulty.

Proximal pelvic muscle weakness can be demonstrated by waddling, a lordotic gait, pelvic or shoulder tilting, and marked lateral thoracic movements on walking.

Proprioceptive sensory loss (posterior columns or roots) is suggested when the patient is ataxic or unsteady in his gait with eyes closed, or when he is unable to see well (as in a dark room), but is not particularly ataxic when he can see.

Tandem Walking (Narrow-based Gait)

The patient is asked to walk as if measuring the floor with the heel placed against the front of the toe with each step. For patients with even minimal cerebellar dysfunction, tandem walking will be impossible to perform well. The examiner should not rush the patient in this test, and should be ready to assist if the patient falters. It is important to be certain that the difficulty the patient shows in tandem gait is not due to vestibular involvement producing drift, or to proximal pelvic muscle weakness.

Heel and Toe Walking

The gait examination provides a convenient time to challenge the powerful leg muscles, often too powerful for examination in recumbency. Plantar flexors (gastrocnemii) are challenged by toe walking, and foot dorsiflexors are challenged by walking on the heels. Since dorsiflexors of the foot are often the earliest muscles to be weakened in hemiparesis or corticospinal system involvement, an early sign is the inability of the patient to keep the ball of the foot as far off the ground on the involved side, as compared to the other side, when heel walking. The ability to keep the heels off the ground equally on toe walking measures plantar flexor strength. Since heel walking also tends to exaggerate the reciprocal arm swing, the symmetry of the swing can be more carefully assessed at this time.

Foot Hopping

The patient is requested to hop continuously first on one foot and then on the other. This assays the strength and coordination of the muscles on one side of the body and is a good screening examination for minimal motor disorder. It represents an excellent survey technique for motor system function. Any inequality in performance demands more careful assessment of leg strength, tone and coordination (see p. 44).

EXAMINATION OF BACK MUSCLES AND SKELETAL STRUCTURES

In addition to examination and palpation of the spinous process of the standing patient for scoliosis, kyphosis, and lordosis, the intraspinous spaces and paravertebral muscles should be palpated for tenderness and spasm accompanying diseases of the spinal cord or nerve root (Fig. 2-1). The back can be percussed for evidence of spinous or intraspinous tenderness or pain. Lateral and forward bending of the trunk, with the legs straight, can often reveal splinting or spasm of the paraspinal muscles in the lumbosacral areas (Fig. 2-2) or provoke sciatic pain in patients with intravertebral disc protrusion or extramedullary cord lesions affecting the posterior roots. It is very important to palpate deeply into the intraspinous spaces of any patient with suspected pathology of the spinal cord, to see if a level of tenderness can be located that may indicate an extramedullary spinal cord lesion. This can be done on the standing, sitting, or supine patient. Detailed palpation of intraspinous spaces may be better accomplished on the

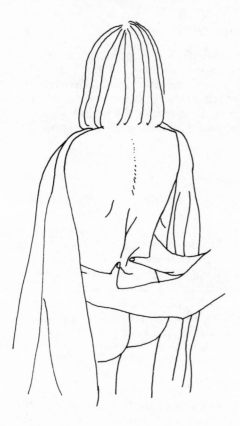

Fig. 2-1. Palpation of paraspinal muscles

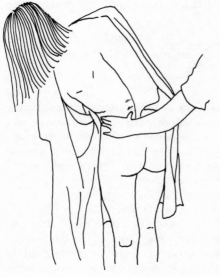

Fig. 2-2. Lateral bending. Note the smooth curve formed by spinal processes and softness of the muscles on the concave side.

supine patient, since the paravertebral muscles will be relaxed and the intraspinous spaces can be opened by forward flexion of the patient's back. While the patient is standing, the sacral notch and hamstring areas can be deeply palpated for evidence of sciatic irritation (Fig. 2-3); the sciatic nerve, in its course, passes through the sciatic notch and the ventral midline of the thigh.

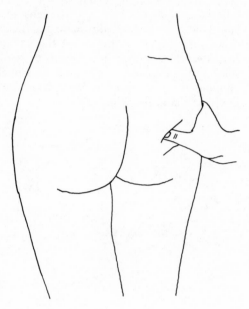

Fig. 2-3. Palpation of the sacral notch for sciatic tenderness

Arm Extension

Maintaining a symmetrical arm posture against gravity (*i.e.*, arms extended with hands supinated or pronated and the eyes closed) requires the integration of many different parts of the motor systems. Subtle disorders may often be revealed. The examiner can add further challenge to strength and coordination by a brisk downward tap on the extended arms.

Corticospinal system dysfunction can be indicated by a slow downward drift of the extended arm. The examiner will also notice easy displacement of the weak arm with a brisk downward tap. With the hands supinated, there will be a tendency for pronation of the hand and flexion of the elbows as the arms are held in continuous extended posture.

Cerebellar dysfunction may be suspected with lateral or upward drift of one arm or increased upward "rebound" of the arm after a brisk downward tap by the examiner.

Extrapyramidal system dysfunction can be suggested by tremor (pill rolling), hyperkinesias (e.g., chorea, athetosis, dystonia, ballism; see p. 12).

Proprioceptive sensory loss in the upper extremities can be manifested by pseudoathetosis (ataxia) of the fingers, a wandering or searching movement of the fingers with the arms extended and the eyes closed.

Muscle weakness due to lower motor neuron or muscle involvement can be suggested either by the difficulty in assuming the extended posture, or fatigue when the arms are in that position for an extended period of time. Specific muscle testing is indicated (see p. 29). Characteristic postures, such as wrist drop or claw hand and atrophy caused by patterns of muscle weakness, point to peripheral nerve lesions.

Leg Extension

Symmetrical leg extension against gravity in either the supine or prone position is of the same significance as arm extension. When the patient is prone with legs flexed 45° at the knees, ballottement of the hamstring tendons (recurrent percussion using the ulnar surface of the examiner's hand) may bring out latent corticospinal weakness manifested by a downward drift of the involved leg (Fig. 2-4). Extension of extended legs in the supine position will fatigue the abdominal muscles quickly. It may be easier for the patient to allow the legs to be flexed at the knees (Fig. 2-5).

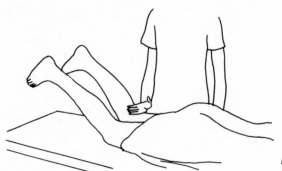

Fig. 2-4. Leg extension, prone with ballottement

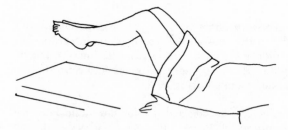

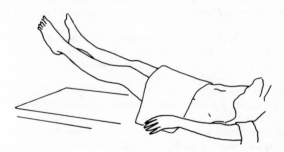

Fig. 2-5. Leg extension, supine

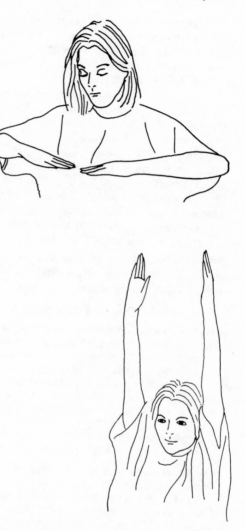

Fig. 2-6. Positions for hyperkinesia

It is important to realize that downward drift of the leg in these tests, especially with ballottement, may indicate corticospinal dysfunction and not necessarily lower motor neuron lesions.

Positions for Detecting Hyperkinesias

The postures illustrated in Figure 2-6 tend to bring out observable hyperkinesias or spontaneous involuntary movements in the upper extremities. While performing formal tests, such as these for hyperkinesia, the examiner must note the movements of all body parts during the examination of the patient. Observations out of the "corner of the eye" while examining the patient are valuable to detect hyperkinetic movements that can often blossom in areas of the body other than the part being formally tested.

It is probably better for the examiner to carefully describe the character of the patient's spontaneous and involuntary movement according to the list below, rather than label them with conventional terms (*e.g.*, chorea, athetosis, dystonia, ballism, asterixis, tremors, myoclonus, spasms, clonus) since these terms have not been defined exactly.

Important Aspects of Movement

Amplitude and rapidity of movements
Distribution of the muscles involved in the movements
Duration of muscle contractions
Direction and rhythm of movement
Effects of willful attempts to stop movements by the patient
Effects of rest, posture holding, and voluntary activity of movements
Effects of fatigue, emotion, sleep, and medication
Extent of muscle involvement; use of the whole muscle or only a part.
  Repetitive use of the same muscle part, or random movements over muscle surface; movement of the joints

Although involuntary movements usually indicate extrapyramidal or basal nuclei involvement (extrapyramidal system), precise localization in anatomical or physiological terms is rarely possible.

CLASSIFICATION OF DYSKINESIAS

Tremor Tremor is a rhythmic oscillation of joints due to alternating contractions of opposing muscles. Tremor is normally present in minute amplitude; it is exaggerated by fatigue, fear, shivering, and in persons with familial or essential tremor. A gross up-and-down tremor called "wing beating" can be seen in patients with Wilson's disease (brought out by the position shown in Fig. 2-6A). With liver disease, a hand-flapping tremor or asterixis can be seen when the arms and wrists are extended forward. It is a quick, recurrent loss and recovery of postural tone in the wrist. Essential or familial tremor often increases in middle age and may mimic the onset of parkinsonism or cerebellar tremor. This tremor can be diminished by alcohol and not by antiparkinsonian drugs. The parkinsonian tremor stops with sleep.

Chorea These involuntary movements are rapid, jerky, irregular, and occur abruptly. Although they are involuntary, the patient may adapt them into purposeful activity (*e.g.*, scratching an ear, putting a hand into a pocket). Mild chorea is hard to distinguish from excessive "fidgets." They are asymmetrical, aggravated by voluntary movement, and, like other extrapyramidal movements, they disappear in sleep. Flicking movements of the fingers, face, tongue, shoulder, knee, and toes can be seen. It is important to observe the entire body. Finger hyperextension at the metacarpophalangeal joint with flexion of the wrist is characteristic.

Athetosis These are slower, writhing, wormlike movements of the distal portions of the extremities. As the hands and feet go through vermicular gyrations, they can assume postures resembling oriental dances. They are aggravated by emotional tension and disappear with sleep.

Dystonia These are powerful, slow movements of principally proximal muscles, twisting the neck (torticollis), the pelvis (tortipelvis), and the back. Patients may demonstrate a very bizarre gait with distortion of walking that can appear hysterical. The characteristic inversion of the foot in plantar flexion, often with extension of the knee, is known as dystonic foot. When the arms are held in the position seen in Figure 2-6B, they may show inward rotation with flexion at the wrist and elbow. Although the back may be normally curved when the patient is erect, it arches strongly when the patient is supine, allowing the examiner to pass his hand under the patient's back. These movements can vary from minimal twists to grotesque disabling postures depending upon the emotional state of the patient. This often leads to psychiatric treatment for "hysteria." They are characteristically aggravated by voluntary motor activity and disappear in sleep.

Ballism Hemiballism, a ballism of the extremities on one side, is seen in persons with partial destruction of the subthalmic nucleus on the contralateral side, usually as a consequence of cerebrovascular occlusion. The patient has wild, continual flail movements of the extremities caused by gross, powerful movements of the proximal muscles; the more distal portions of the extremity follow in a passive whiplike manner. Unless sufficient precautions are taken, the patient's movements can easily cause a fracture of the arm or leg against bedrails. The patient can die of exhaustion if the movements are not controlled.

Akinesia This is a most crippling, yet often unnoticed, sign of extrapyramidal involvement. It is the absence of spontaneous motor activities that we all perform automatically. Even though the patient is not weak, the initiation of muscle activity is an effort in akinesia. Akinesia can be further suggested by a masked, emotionless face. Gaze movement of the eyes to the right, left, or upward can occur without the usual associated movement of the head or brows. The patient sits motionless, devoid of the usual small constant muscle activities characteristic of the normal human. It is the antithesis of *hyper*kinesia mentioned above. It is often associated with flexed postures of neck, trunk, arms, and legs.

Parkinsons

Myoclonic Movements These are quick, violent, repetitive movements of an extremity usually triggered by activity and involving proximal muscles. Their clonic, seizurelike appearance is obvious. These movements can be seen in patients with diffuse cortical lesions of the cerebrum or cerebellum, and with grey matter lesions of the spinal cord. They are probably not of extrapyramidal origin. They can occur spontaneously and are often part of seizure phenomena.

The Finger-to-Nose Test Coordination of the muscles in the arm can be tested by asking the patient to touch his nose with the index finger of each hand, starting with the arm in the extended position. The patient should be asked to do this initially with the eyes closed and then with the eyes open (Fig. 2-7). The examiner should note whether there is an improvement in performance when the eyes are open.

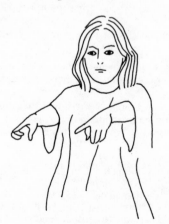 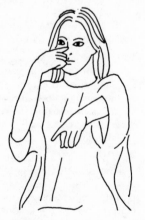

Fig. 2-7. Finger-to-nose test, performed with eyes closed and then open

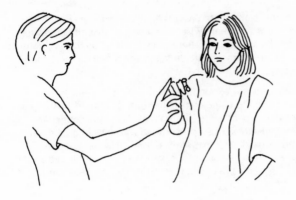

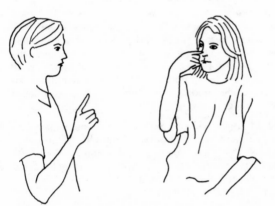

Fig. 2-8. Finger-to-nose-to-finger test. As the patient moves her finger back and forth from her nose to the examiner's, the examiner changes finger position.

The Finger-to-Nose-to-Finger Test A further challenge to the coordination of the arm muscles can be made by asking the patient, eyes open, to alternately touch the examiner's finger held at approximately arms length form the patient, and then his own nose. As this is repeated, the examiner moves his finger about into many different positions, some almost beyond the patient's reach (Fig. 2-8).

In these examinations, two phenomena may be sought that indicate cerebellar dysfunction. They can occur separately or together.

1. Dysmetria (or disordered measurements of motion in space) causes arm movement in an inappropriate direction and over-correction movements as the finger attempts to touch the tip of the nose (Fig. 2-9).
2. Intention (action) tremor is a rapid oscillating tremor of the finger that usually develops just prior to reaching the nose or the examiner's finger (Fig. 2-10). It often increases with the proximity of the finger to the target. This tremor can be minimal.

Both phenomena cause disordered movement in a horizontal plane.

If the dysmetria on finger-to-nose examination is produced only when the patient's eyes are closed, or if it is markedly worsened when the eyes are closed, this suggests a proprioceptive sensory loss of information to the cerebellum due to peripheral nerve, cord, or brain stem lesions. Vision can provide adequate sensory feedback to the cerebellum and can correct motor disability due to proprioceptive sensory loss. This

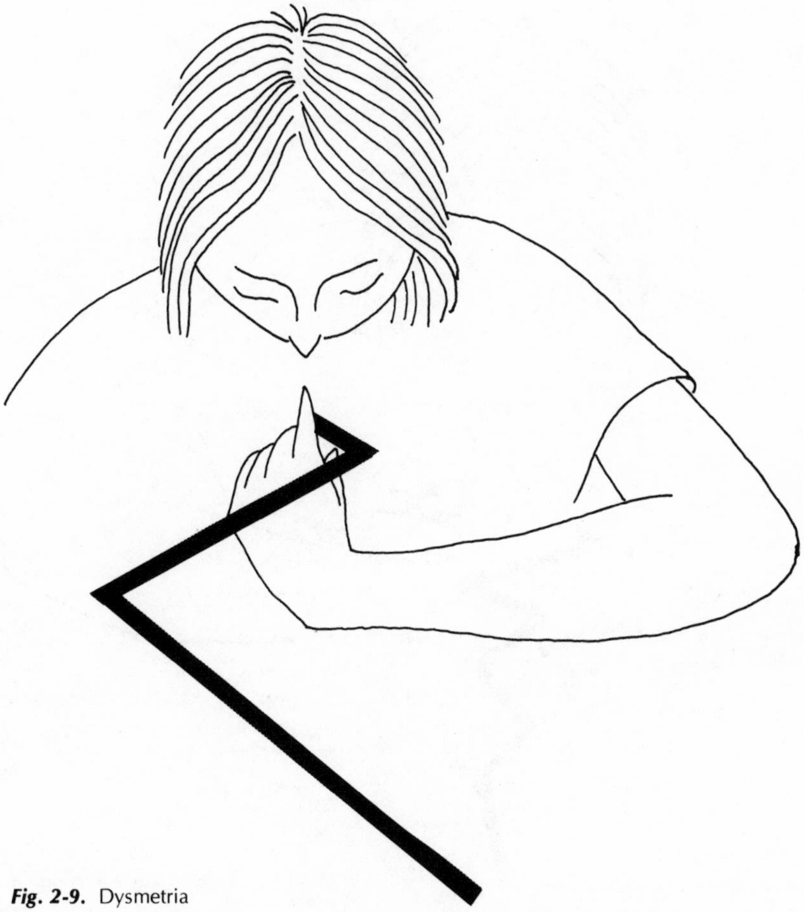

Fig. 2-9. Dysmetria

phenomenon can be seen even when proprioceptive sensation is intact on formal sensory examination if the so-called "unconscious proprioceptive pathways" (spinocerebellar) are involved.

Muscle weakness of the arms may simulate dysmetria since inadequate strength affects timing and coordination of the involved muscles. This can usually be differentiated from a cerebellar disorder by findings on the rest of the neurological examination. However, if the examiner resists the arm movement by placing a mild restraint with his fingers against the patient's moving arm or leg, the dysmetria will diminish in patients with cerebellar dysfunction and be intensified in those with weakness.

Extrapyramidal or parkinsonian tremor, unlike cerebellar intention tremor, usually does not increase as the nose is approached (action tremor); the tremor may diminish. This tremor is usually present when the arms are held extended (postural tremor) unlike the cerebellar type of tremor.

With lesions of the superior cerebellar peduncle or those in the region of the red nucleus, the cerebellar tremor can have a postural component seen when the arms are extended. This postural or parkinsonian tremor blends into an intention tremor on movement of the finger to the nose, and ends again as a postural tremor as the patient attempts to hold the finger against the nose ("rubral" tremor).

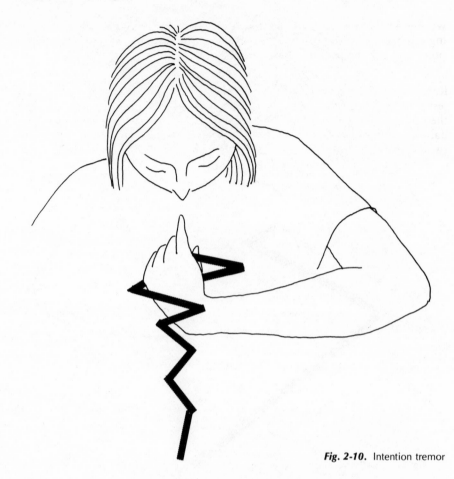

Fig. 2-10. Intention tremor

Heel-to-Toe-Test In this examination, as in the finger-to-nose examination, the physician looks for dymetria and tremor. It is important to remember that the leg is considerably more clumsy and less skillful than the arms, and even in the normal patient there may be some evidence of dysmetric performance. The examiner asks the patient to place his heel on his knee and slide it down the shin to the foot (Fig. 2-11).

Decomposition of movement is often described in this test for cerebellar lesions. The hip and the knee flex at inappropriate rates and, as a result, the heel usually shoots well above and beyond the knee. Corrective movements have to be made to eventually put the heel on the knee. There is no reason to separate this phenomenon from dysmetria; both probably represent the same process. Intention (action) tremor can also be seen as the heel moves down the shin.

Toe-to-Finger Test This is a more challenging cerebellar test for the lower extremities. The examiner should place his finger in such a way that the patient has to bend the knee in order to touch the finger with the great toe. Here,

finger
like nose to
finger to

weakness of the muscles may produce a very poor performance, falsely suggesting cerebellar difficulty. Again, the examiner can move his finger from point to point and ask the patient to follow with the toe.

Rapid Alternating Movements (Diadochokinesia) The patient can perform this test by tapping the thighs with both hands, alternately on the palmar surface and then on the dorsal surface, or by tapping one hand in the same manner on the palm of the other. A less difficult and less sensitive test is to ask the patient to twist the wrists alternately back and forth as if screwing in overhead light bulbs.

Characteristics of Cerebellar Dysdiadochokinesia

Performance is unrhythmical but rapid.

√ Accuracy of hand placement varies with each tap.

Excursion of the hand is inappropriately large and varied for the maneuver re- ? quested. The patient usually does not show full supination of the hand.

Left and right hands are not well coordinated when working together.

Frequently, the elbows and shoulders are also brought into exaggerated movement as they assist the hands in their performance.

With corticospinal or extrapyramidal disease, the performance of the patient may be correct in terms of placement and rhythm but is labored and slow. Arthritis can also affect this performance.

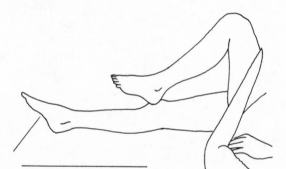

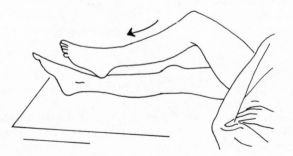

Fig. 2-11. Heel-to-toe test

Rapid Alternating Movements of the Foot   The patient is asked to tap the ball of his foot rapidly against a flat surface. With the patient in a supine position, the examiner can offer the palm of his hand as a surface. The sitting patient can tap his foot on the floor. This examination cannot be performed standing. Cerebellar disease produces an uncoordinated, unrhythmical performance, and corticospinal or extrapyramidal disease produces a labored or slow performance.

Check   The examiner asks the patient to pull his fist toward his own face as hard as he can while the examiner restrains it at the wrist. Without warning, the examiner quickly opens his fingers and releases the wrist. In the normal person, the fist stops abruptly because the previously relaxed antagonist triceps muscle suddenly contracts and "checks" the rapid advance of the released isometrically contracted biceps. In cerebellar disease, such "check" does not occur quickly enough, and the patient might hit his face if it is not protected by the examiner's other hand (Fig. 2-12). There are many variations of this "cerebellar" test.

Sitting Up   Sitting up from a supine position requires coordination of the bilateral axial and extremity muscles for a smooth performance.

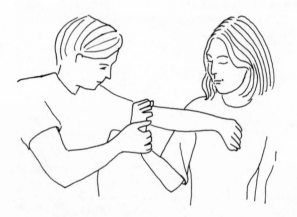

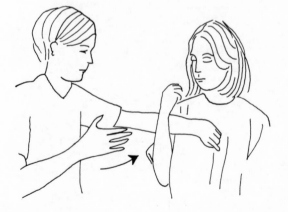

Fig. 2-12. Testing for check. Note the examiner's arm protecting the patient's face.

In patients with cerebellar dysfunctions, the legs can fly in the air, and the trunk moves in a jerky, ataxic fashion. The patient can sit only if the examiner holds down his feet. In patients with corticospinal tract dysfunction, the examiner may note a premature and greater elevation of the leg on the suspected hemiparetic side (trunk-thigh sign). Also, the shoulder on the opposite side may be seen to elevate earlier.

Handedness The dominant hand is usually the hand chosen by the patient for writing, dialing the phone, pulling a cork from a bottle, dealing cards, cutting with scissors, and throwing. The size of the thumbnail, especially the breadth of the "U" at the base, is larger in the dominant hand.

Careful inquiry may reveal hand preference determined in childhood by parental training, or injury to an arm or hand. Evidence of ambidexterity in the patient or relatives, or left-handed relatives of a right-handed patient, may suggest that the preferred hand for writing in the patient is not contralateral to the hemisphere for language communication. Such concern is warranted in the evaluation of hemisphere lesions associated with communication disorders (aphasia; see Chapter 8). Evidence is lacking to support the theory that eye or foot preference or other factors are reliably related to the hemisphere concerned with communication.

For convenience here, we will refer to the average or commonest situation in which the left hemisphere is responsible for language and symbolism including handwriting, and the right hemisphere deals with temporal and spatial phenomena. As this is true in nearly all right-handed persons, and probably for the majority of left-handers as well, the chances are great that most patients, regardless of handedness, have left cerebral language dominance.

Praxis Praxis is the ability to perform the complex, voluntary motor skills normally expected for the individual's age, training, or capabilities. Implicit in the term is the need for cortical integration in the production of the activity. Praxic skills can be tested by such actions as the sequential tapping of each finger-tip by the thumb, buttoning, using a toothbrush or comb, mimicking, or gesturing. Performance of charades without concrete objects (*e.g.*, drinking from an imaginary glass provided by the examiner) provides more of a challenge for praxic skills. The actual presence of an object, such as a toothbrush or a glass, may cause the skill to be automatically or reflexly performed without requiring higher cortical skills. Asking the patient to mimic hand-tapping patterns, with progressively more complex rhythms and varieties of hand and finer configuration, can provide greater challenge to praxis.

Apraxia, implying cortical motor involvement, can only be suspected when there is no significant weakness or incoordination in the extremities tested. Buccofacial apraxia and apraxia of gait are common. The former is seen in the patient who cannot voluntarily, on command, protrude the tongue or purse the lips. Yet, he will make these movements automatically when his lips are dry or if a hard candy is placed on the lips. A patient with apraxia of gait has difficulty walking voluntarily on the examiner's command. Nevertheless, he might walk quite well when he is not thinking about it. For example, he might walk without impairment to the bathroom automatically and without thinking. If you ask the patient with apraxia of gait to alternately place one foot in front of the other, he will be able to walk.

Apraxia usually implies a lesion in the premotor cortex of the dominant hemi- ✷

sphere (see communication testing, Chapter 8). However, apraxia can also be seen with parietal cortex lesions as well as lesions of the corpus callosum. These locations also emphasize the artificial dichotomy between the motor and sensory systems. Recalled sensory patterns and sensory feedback are basic to controlled motor performance.

Dressing and Undressing This is a routine act in which skill is expected of everyone. It should be a reasonably quick and dexterous performance. The examiner may ask the patient to button or unbutton with only one hand to observe the skill of each.

This action can be readily observed as the patient prepares for examination. Clumsy, akinetic, ataxic performance can provide clues to apraxia, upper motor neuron weakness, lower motor neuron weakness, and cerebellar or extrapyramidal dysfunction. The examiner's conclusion depends on the character of the performance and other findings in the examination.

Handwriting This is a complex motor performance requiring cooperation of many muscles in fine rapid patterns.

This performance depends upon integration of motor and sensory systems at all levels including the cortex. Although there is much individual variation unique to the patient, there are some abnormal patterns of diagnostic value in the motor examination. For example, patients with cerebellar system dysfunction display an ataxic, incoordinated, ever-widening and rising script as the hand moves across the page. The script is increasingly deformed by dysmetric movements of the pencil (macrographia). In extrapyramidal disease, the patient produces a tight, squared, jagged script that becomes smaller in size and more cramped as the hand crosses the page (micrographia). If the patient shows left-sided neglect of the page on writing or a misalignment of the writing angle, a minor hemisphere lesion may be indicated.

Drawing The patient should be asked to draw basic forms or shapes (*e.g.*, a clock with its face and numbers, a daisy, or a house). The patient can also be asked to copy nonsense patterns produced by the examiner.

Drawing assesses the patient's ability to communicate with graphic symbolism. However, drawing also tests spatial orientation and muscle coordination. Distortions or an inability to draw can be seen in patients with parietal lobe lesions, particularly if a left (or dominant) parietal lobe lesion is deep enough to interfere with callosal fibers from the right (nondominant) parietal lobe. Deeper lesions near the optic radiations can show drawing distortions that represent a hemianopic disorder (*i.e.*, half the figure is incomplete or distorted). Left sided inattention to the page or to the figure in the drawing indicates right hemisphere pathology, particularly in the parietal lobe. Gross over-simplification and primitive construction in drawing is frequently associated with lesions in the left hemisphere. The loss of perspective or disturbances in the relations between different parts of a drawing has been called "constructional apraxia."

Finger Dexterity Tests Tapping the index finger on the distal joint of the thumb is a simple, valuable test for manual dexterity (Fig. 2-13).

Corticospinal system dysfunction produces a slowed performance and an increased movement of the thumb to obtain closure between the finger and the thumb.

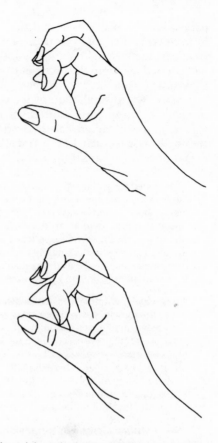

Fig. 2-13. Finger dexterity test

Extrapyramidal dysfunction produces a slow, labored, akinetic performance. Cerebellar system dysfunction produces a nonrhythmical performance with over- and under-shooting of the joint by the tapping finger.

Rapid, sequential touching of each finger to the thumb is another convenient test, especially if there is no opportunity to see the patient demonstrate manual skills on dressing or undressing.

Muscle Tone

In the clinical examination, muscle tone can be defined as the resistance offered by muscle to a stretch accomplished by passive movement of a joint. The examiner must be certain that the patient's muscles are relaxed so that tone is not affected by voluntary muscle contraction. It is important that the student test muscle tone consistently in all patients so that he learns the "feel" of normal tone.

Testing of tone is a valuable and often neglected part of the examination. Tone should be elicited in the neck, arms, and legs. The examiner should move methodically from distal to proximal extremity. Neck muscle tone can be felt when the patient passively flexes and extends the head, or when the supine patient lifts the head off the bed and lets it drop. Muscle rigidity may cause the head to remain elevated or drop slowly (head-dropping test). To test the extremities, the examiner should hold the extremity just proximal to the joints being tested and note the laxity of distal joint movement when the extremity is shaken. The examiner can also flex and extend joints passively, again noting any resistance. Rapid supination of the patient's forearm may bring out increased pronator tone, an early and sensitive sign of spasticity. When the patient is supine, a rapid lift and release of the relaxed leg, with the examiner's hand under the popliteal space, can demonstrate the degree of quadriceps muscle tone by the extent of foot elevation; increased tone prevents easy flexion of the knee.

Reduced tone, flaccidity, or hypotonia, can be seen in patients with lower motor neuron diseases involving either the anterior horn cell, motor root, or peripheral nerve, and is found occasionally in patients with muscle diseases. Hypotonia may be associated with cerebellar lesions. Increased tone (hypertonia) is characteristically found in upper motor neuron disease (corticospinal, pyramidal) and disease of the basal ganglia (extrapyramidal system). Often these two varieties of hypertonia may be distinguished in the examination of the patient and help differentiate corticospinal or pyramidal dysfunction from extrapyramidal dysfunction as follows:

Spasticity (Pyramidal or Corticospinal Dysfunction) The hypertonia is greater when the joint is passively moved in one direction and less when moved in the other. Characteristically, hypertonicity on extension of the elbow or wrist is greater than on flexion, and the reverse is true in the knee and ankle. Hypertonicity increases as the muscles are passively stretched or lengthened (usually elbow extension and knee flexion). Occasionally, hypertonicity increases to the point where the hypertonicity may suddenly dissolve and the muscle extends the rest of the way with ease ("clasp-knife" phenomenon). Spasticity may show differences in its pattern depending on the location of the upper motor neuron lesion and the posture of the patient.

Rigidity (Basal Ganglia or Extrapyramidal System Dysfunction) Here the resistance to passive joint movement is equal in both extension and flexion and unchanging in intensity as the joint goes through its complete range ("plastic rigidity"). The tendons on both the flexor and extensor sides of the joint maintain tension during all ranges of flexion and extension. Frequently, an underlying tremor can be felt against a background of rigidity on passive motion, giving the sensation that the joint is passing over cogs as in a cog-and-rachet movement (cogwheel rigidity). This is usually seen in patients with parkinsonian rigidity.

Gegenhalten (Bilateral Frontal Lobe Lesions) This is an exaggeration of tone in the muscles being passively stretched, giving the appearance of voluntary opposition to the movement by the patient. For example, when the examiner attempts passive elbow extension, it appears as if the patient is actively flexing the elbow.

Decorticate Spasticity Decorticate spasticity, seen in patients with diffuse, usually subcortical, hemispheric lesions, is characterized by flexor posturing of the arms and extension of the legs and feet with strong adduction of the legs.

Decerebrate Spasticity In decerebrate spasticity the legs are also in extension and adduction, but the upper extremities are in extension and internal rotation. Medullary or spinal spasticity involves primarily the lower extremities and is predominantly extensor. Here, walking is on the tips of the toes ("digitigrade walk"). In certain circumstances, especially with bladder infection or skin ulcerations, the spasticity in the lower extremities may become flexor in pattern.

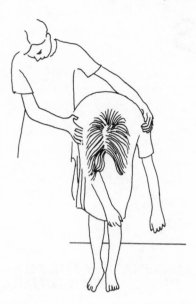

Fig. 2-14. Estimating pendulousness in the arms

in affected?

Muscle Tone with Contralateral Motor Activity Minimal, subclinical, or questionable extrapyramidal rigidity can often be increased when a patient performs a repetitive movement (*e.g.*, tapping the hand or foot) with the extremity contralateral to the one being examined. This does not cause increased tone in the normal patient or in those with spasticity.

Tests for Pendulousness Unless the patient can fully relax the muscles, these *due to hypotonia* tests are invalid. An increased and persisting to-and-fro swinging at a joint ("pendulousness"), beyond what can be expected normally, is seen in patients with cerebellar lesions. When the patient is sitting, this may be noted in free swinging of the knee after the knee jerk is elicited. In the standing patient, pendulousness may be indicated by increased swinging of the arms when the shoulders are shaken in the horizontal plane by the examiner (Fig. 2-14). Pendulousness can also be estimated by the ease with which the arms, hanging by the sides, can be flipped away from the hips. Decreased tone can also be detected when the examiner holds the patient's forearms vertically and notes the degree of flexion at the wrist of the dangling hands. The examiner must determine whether any manifestation of reduced tone is due to a lower motor neuron disorder, muscle disease, or cerebellar involvement.

3

EXAMINATION OF INDIVIDUAL MUSCLES

EXAMINATION FOR MUSCLE ATROPHY AND NORMAL BODY CONTOURS

The earliest clue to muscle atrophy, seen in lower motor neuron or muscle disease, is the loss of body contours that are produced by normal muscle bulk. Not only can individual muscle involvement be detected, but the overall pattern of muscle involvement can be assayed. This is important in considering whether weakness is of myogenic or neurogenic origin, and in making the differentiation between focal and diffuse disease processes. Muscle hypertrophy can also be detected by carefully examining all body contours; thus, it is important to inspect the entire body carefully when necessary. The student should familiarize himself with the contribution each muscle makes to body contours; the examiner should become familiar with the anatomical contours produced by the muscles of even poorly muscled patients. Normal or abnormal distribution of fat may obscure these landmarks on the trunk and proximal extremities.

MUSCLE PERCUSSION FOR MYOTATIC IRRITABILITY AND FASCICULATION

Myotatic irritability is a contraction of muscle bundles when they are directly percussed by the hammer or fingers. This is seen in patients with chronic diseases, malnutrition, and lower motor neuron disease (anterior horn cell and motor root). The normally present myotatic irritability of the deltoid muscle must not be considered pathological.

Fasciculations are small, flickering, nonrhythmical contractions of muscle fascicles seen only as a brief dimpling or rippling under the skin. This can be difficult to see in obese patients. Fasciculation occurs spontaneously but can often be elicited by tapping the muscle several times with a hammer or fingers. Fasciculation is not an immediate result of the percussion, but occurs spontaneously in the seconds following the multiple percussions. Its visibility can be enhanced by tangential lighting of the body surfaces under examination. Fasciculations can sometimes be heard with a stethoscope in fully relaxed muscles.

Fasciculations usually indicate the presence of anterior horn cell disease or, less commonly, motor root or, rarely, peripheral nerve dysfunction. Fasciculations are seen also in electrolyte disturbances and in myopathies due to hyperthyroidism and polymyositis. Fasciculations of pathologic significance should not be confused with "benign" fasciculations nearly everyone notices around the eyes, in the calves, and in the fingers. These are usually large in size and are often felt before they are seen. Benign fasciculations can move a joint or lid and often are aggravated by fatigue and tension. All varieties of fasciculations, normal and pathological, are aggravated by cold. These facts can be helpful in the examination of the patient. The pathological significance of observed fasciculations in the patient must be verified by such clinical neurophysiologic investigations as electromyography.

MUSCLE PALPATION

The normal consistency or turgor of muscles on palpation should be learned as a sensory experience so that abnormalities can be noted in the examination of patients. In patients with muscular dystrophy and polymyositis, for example, muscles may have a fibrous, tough consistency. Palpation may also reveal muscle tenderness.

EXAMINATION FOR MYOTONIC PHENOMENA

Myotonia is an involuntary repetitive discharge of muscle fibers causing prolonged muscle contraction. It may be elicited by strong and sudden voluntary muscle activity on the part of the patient. It is characteristically elicited during examination of the grip. The patient is asked to grip something small (*e.g.*, one or two fingers) very tightly and then instructed to suddenly open the hand. In cases of myotonia, the patient cannot release and open the hand rapidly. During the attempted rapid opening, the myotonic's hand shows hyperextension of the distal finger joints. Percussion of skeletal muscle may also demonstrate myotonic contraction, most characteristically seen with percussion of the thenar eminence and the tongue. In myotonia, percussion of such muscle bellies causes a visible humping, which in turn is caused by localized muscle contraction and slow relaxation.

The phenomenon of myotonia is found in several diseases of muscle. The presence of myotonia causes labored hand opening due to continued contraction of the flexor muscles. Such rare conditions as myotonia congentia may be associated with diffuse myotonia. Myotonia can also be seen occasionally in other conditions (e.g., polymyositis, periodic paralysis, motor neuron diseases, and hypothyroid myopathy). It tends to diminish with repeated activity and is aggravated by cold.

MEASUREMENT OF MUSCLE ATROPHY

The circumference of a limb is due largely to its muscle bulk. Measurement can serve as an objective estimate of muscle atrophy. The measurement of limb circumference must be made at homologous points on opposite extremities where the circumference is at its maximum. This is ensured by measuring at a fixed distance from a bony landmark (*e.g.,* the patellar notch or olecranon). The landmark and distance should be noted in the examiner's written report. The examiner should ensure that the tightness of the tape is the same on both sides. Measurement of limb circumference with right and left comparison may document the presence of significant atrophy. A difference of two centimeters in limb circumference between sides can be considered significant. Such documentation allows for accurate assessment of change on subsequent examination.

OBJECTIVE TESTS OF MUSCLE STRENGTH

Testing the strength of the patient's muscles is one of the least objective and least reliable portions of the neurological examination. Some objectivity of measurement is needed to assay the degree of functional impairment, and to determine on subsequent examinations whether the patient is improving or worsening. This can be provided by using gravity as a constant source of pull against the patient's muscles. In this manner, the following muscles, as examples, can be tested.

Tibialis Anterior (Heel Walking) The examiner notes the patient's ability to keep the ball of the foot the same distance off the ground on both sides during walking. This is a particularly valuable test for early corticospinal pyramidal dysfunction, since the dorsiflexors of the foot are almost always involved early in minimal hemiplegia. These muscles can also be tested by asking the patient to stand on the heels, both unilaterally and bilaterally, for a period of time.

Gastrocnemii (Toe Walking) The examiner notes the patient's ability to keep both heels the same distance off the ground while walking. These muscles can be tested also by asking the patient to stand on the toes of one or both feet for a period of time.

Gluteals When standing, the patient is asked to raise a knee high in the air; the contralateral gluteus medius keeps the hip elevated on the side of the raised knee (Fig. 3-1). Contralateral gluteal weakness is manifested by a dropping of the hip on the side of the raised knee. The comparative height of the hips is best estimated by placing the hands on the top of both iliac crests. This is an excellent test of early weakness in a muscle group that is very powerful and hard to examine.

Proximal Pelvic Muscles—Bilateral To rise from a chair and sit in a chair gracefully requires the combined action of gluteals and quadriceps. The patient should be asked to keep arms crossed on the chest so that they will not automatically assist him in rising from the chair. With the supine patient, elevation of the straight leg requires combined iliopsoas and quadriceps function. An early corticospinal lesion will manifest itself by a slow, downward drift of the leg on the involved side. Elevating both legs simultaneously for a period of time is a challenge to these muscles and will expose minimal weakness.

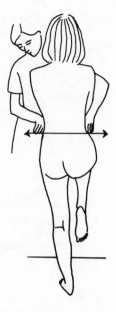

Fig. 3-1. Stabilization of the *right* iliac crest by action of the *left* gluteus medius.

Proximal Pelvic Muscles—Unilateral Stepping up on a chair or stool utilizes gluteal and quadriceps muscles of the leg and allows a comparison between the left and right sides.

Bilateral Proximal Pectoral Muscles Holding the arms outstretched horizontally from the shoulder for a prolonged period of time requires deltoid and trapezius action. The time the patient can hold this position is a relatively objective measurement of strength. The examiner can further challenge the strength of the proximal pectoral muscles by pushing down on the arms at more and more distal positions on the arms (Fig. 3-2)

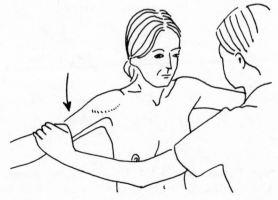

Fig. 3-2. Deltoid. As in most muscle tests, the contraction of the muscle belly can be seen.

MUSCLE SURVEY FOR PATTERNS OF WEAKNESS

The examiner should develop a rapid survey technique for testing skeletal muscle strength. If the survey reveals evidence of weakness, more detailed testing is required to determine the specific muscles involved. The pattern or combination of muscles involved can indicate to the examiner the anatomical position of the lesion (*i.e.,* cerebral hemisphere, brain stem, cord segment, motor root, plexus, peripheral nerves, or a combination of these) and whether the lesion is diffuse or focal.

A scale of 0 to 5 can be used to attempt an objective record of muscle strength. Five implies normal muscle strength. Four indicates somewhat reduced muscle strength. Three implies an inability to overcome the examiner's resistance but enough strength to move the extremity against the downward pull of gravity. Two indicates enough strength to produce movement if the pull of gravity is eliminated. One implies visible muscle contraction but insufficient to produce movement. Zero implies no evidence of muscle contraction. It is important for the examiner to develop a technique that is constant for him from patient to patient so that he has an awareness of "normal." He must be sure that he is not inadvertently testing nearby muscles that can produce movements similar to those of the muscles under investigation. The examiner should note the bulging or visible contraction of the muscles tested, or the contraction of the muscle's tendon whenever possible. Contracting muscles can also be palpated during examination.

The following tests offer a routine that the examiner can modify or abridge to suit the patient's problem. The examiner should be able to test arm and leg muscles with the patient in either the supine or sitting position.

Neck Flexors—C1-C4 These are normally not very strong muscles (Fig. 3-3). (The sternocleidomastoid muscles are innervated by the cranial nerve XI; their test is shown in the cranial nerve section on p. 118.) Note that the examiner puts a supporting hand behind the patient.

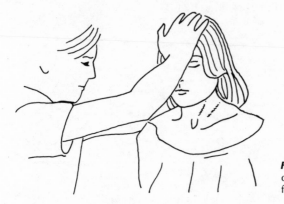

Fig. 3-3. Neck flexors. The examiner's other hand is against the patient's back for stabilization.

Neck Extensors—C1-C4 These muscles, by contrast, are quite strong (Fig. 3-4). The examiner supports the patient with the other hand against the chest.

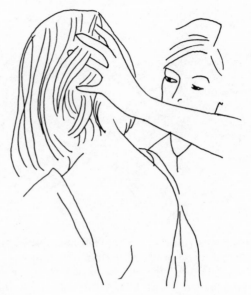

Fig. 3-4. Neck extensors. The examiner's other hand is against the patient's chest for stabilization.

Upper Trapezius Muscles—Accessory Nerve, C3-C4 These are very strong muscles. The examiner should not be able to depress the patient's shoulder (Fig. 3-5).

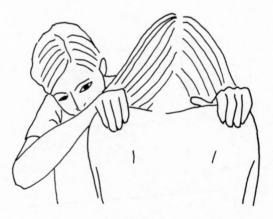

Fig. 3-5. Upper trapezius muscles

Rhomboids—Dorsal Scapular Nerve, C4-C5 With the fist at the hip, the patient resists the examiner's attempt to rotate the elbows forward by externally rotating his shoulders (Fig. 3-6). The contracting muscle mass can be seen between the medial edge of the scapula and the spinous processes of the thoracic vertebrae.

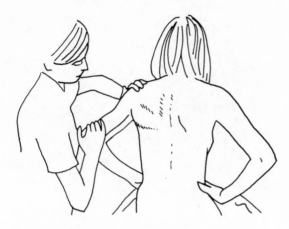

Fig. 3-6. Rhomboids. The examiner attempts to push patient's elbow forward against resistance.

Serratus Anterior—Long Thoracic Nerve, C5-C7 Muscular weakness is indicated by an outward flaring and an upward winging of the medial edge of the scapula when the patient pushes against a wall or the examiner pushes against the patient's extended arm (Fig. 3-7). Both the serratus anterior and the trapezius hold the scapula to the thoracic cage. Winging of the scapula can be seen with weakness of either muscle group. However, the weakness can be differentiated by an awareness of each muscle's action. Weakness of the trapezius causes outward rotation of the scapula. Weakness of the serratus anterior causes inward rotation of the scapula and flaring of the medial border.

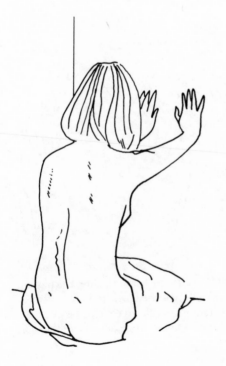

Fig. 3-7. Serratus anterior

Latissimus Dorsi—Subscapular Nerve, C6-C8   The examiner lifts his horizontally oriented fingers high into the patient's axilla to feel the contraction of the muscle tendon during coughing. The arms must be dependent and relaxed. The muscle can often be observed contracting on the patient's back.

Pectoralis Group—Pectoral Nerves, C5-T1   With an externally rotated shoulder and flexed elbow, the patient resists the examiner's attempt to push the elbows externally or outward. The degree of elbow elevation determines whether the test emphasis is on the upper pectoral (Fig. 3-8) or lower pectoral groups (Fig. 3-9). Another method is to ask the patient to forcibly press the hands together in an exaggerated prayer position. The pectoral muscles can be seen to contract bilaterally and can be compared (Fig. 3-10).

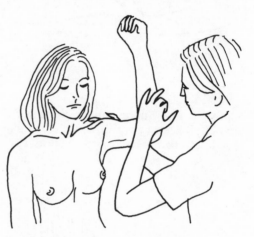

Fig. 3-8. Upper pectoral muscles. The examiner attempts to rotate the patient's arm outward against resistance.

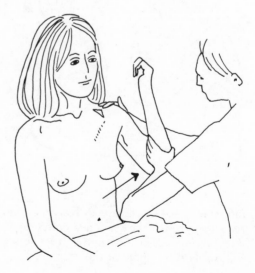

Fig. 3-9. Lower pectoral muscles

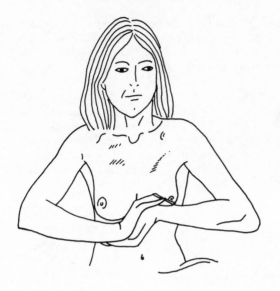

Fig. 3-10. Pectoralis group

Supraspinatus—Suprascapular Nerve, C5 The patient attempts to abduct his elbows pinned at his sides by the examiner's hands. The contraction of the muscle can be observed in the suprascapular space (Fig. 3-11).

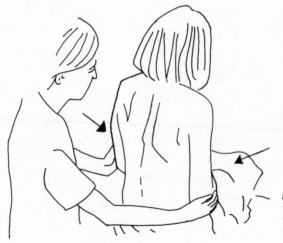

Fig. 3-11. Supraspinatus. The patient attempts to abduct elbows from her side. The examiner looks for the bulge of the supraspinatus.

Infraspinatus—Suprascapular Nerve, C5-C6 With elbows held tight to his side, the patient resists the examiner's attempt to rotate his forearms together in the midline (Fig. 3-12). The muscle can be seen contracting in the infraspinatus space below the spine of the scapula.

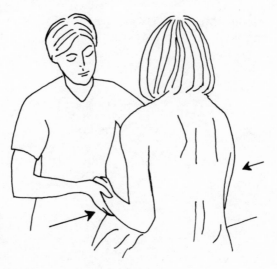

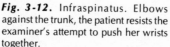

Fig. 3-12. Infraspinatus. Elbows against the trunk, the patient resists the examiner's attempt to push her wrists together.

Deltoid—Axillary Nerve, C5-C6 Arm abduction beyond 45° is essential to test this muscle. The examiner attempts to depress the abducted arm (see Fig. 3-2). The deltoid can be clearly seen. Strength can be quantitated by noting how far distally the examiner must place his hands on the patient's arm to easily overcome the deltoids.

Triceps—Radial Nerve, C6-C8 The patient attempts to extend his elbow against resistance by the examiner (Fig. 3-13). The triceps is best tested with the elbow flexed. The more the elbow is extended, the more difficult it is to overcome the strength of the triceps. Exact strength can never be determined unless the examiner is able to overcome the patient's muscle.

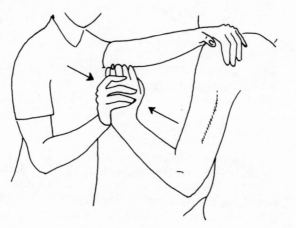

Fig. 3-13. Triceps

Biceps—Musculocutaneous Nerve, C5-C7   The biceps is the principal flexor of the elbow when the wrist is *supinated* (Fig. 3-14).

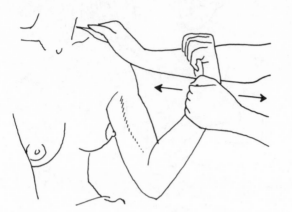

Fig. 3-14. Biceps

Brachioradialis—Radial Nerve, C5-C6   This muscle is the principal flexor of the arm when the wrist is semipronated (Fig. 3-15). The tendon can be seen in the forearm.

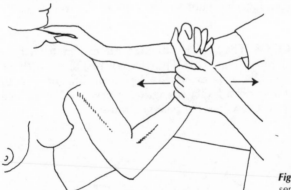

Fig.3-15. Brachioradialis. Note the semipronated wrist.

Wrist Extensors—Radial Nerve, C6-C8   The examiner attempts to depress the patient's extended wrist while supporting the patient's forearm. This is a strong muscle and is equal bilaterally despite hand dominance. It is important in skeletal muscle surveys because of its early involvement in pyramidal hemiplegia or upper motor neuron lesions.

Wrist Flexors—Median Nerve, C6-T1   The examiner attempts to overcome the patient's flexed wrist in the same manner.

Flexor Digitorum Sublimis—Median Nerve, C7-T1   It is important that the examiner ensure fixation of the proximal phalanx and extension at the distal phalangeal joint (Fig. 3-16). The action of this muscle is to flex an interphalangeal joint.

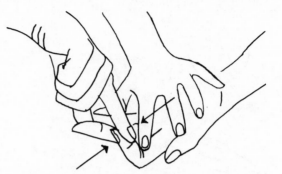

Fig. 3-16. Flexor digitorum sublimis

Flexor Digitorum Profundus—Median Nerve, C8-T1 Here the patient's hand should be positioned to test flexion only at the distal interphalangeal joint (Fig. 3-17). Note that the examiner's hand is extending the middle interphalangeal joint.

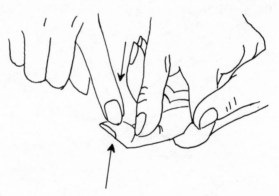

Fig. 3-17. Flexor digitorum profundus

Flexor Pollicis Longus—Median Nerve, C8-T1 This is the flexor of the distal thumb joint (Fig. 3-18).

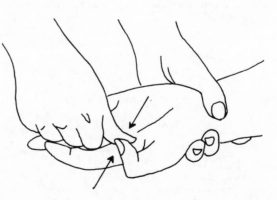

Fig. 3-18. Flexor pollicis longus

Abductor Pollicis Brevis—Median Nerve, C8-T1 The patient is abducting (or elevating) the thumb at right angles to the plane of the palm. The examiner's finger is pressing downward (Fig. 3-19).

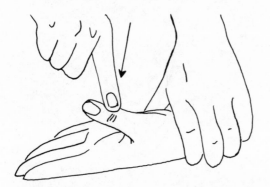

Fig. 3-19. Abductor pollicis brevis

Opponens Pollicis—Median Nerve, C8-T1 The examiner asks the patient to touch the base of the little finger with her thumb and resist the examiner's attempts to pull it away (Fig. 3-20). When this muscle is very weak, the patient's thumbnail rotates to a position parallel to the plane of the palm.

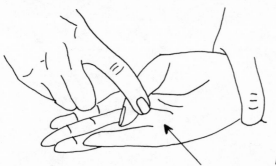

Fig. 3-20. Opponens pollicis

Thumb Extensors—Radial Nerve, C7-C8 The examiner attempts to overcome the extended thumb (Fig. 3-21). If other distal muscles are weak, the hand should be fully supported on a firm surface so that only the thumb extensor is being tested.

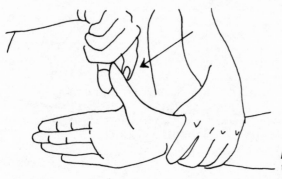

Fig. 3-21. Thumb extensors. These tendons can be easily seen.

Abductor Digiti Minimi—Ulnar Nerve, C8-T1 The examiner attempts to overcome the abducted little finger; the patient's hand is prone on a flat surface (Fig. 3-22).

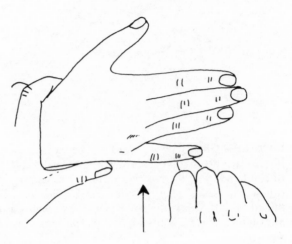

Fig. 3-22. Abductor digiti minimi

Adductor Digiti Minimi—Ulnar Nerve, C8-T1 The patient resists the examiner's attempt to pull the little finger from the hand laterally (Fig. 3-23).

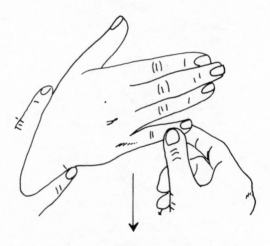

Fig. 3-23. Adductor digiti minimi

Adductor Pollicis—Ulnar Nerve, C8-T1 The patient's thumb is tightly held to the lateral surface of the first finger, and the examiner attempts to pull it away (Fig. 3-24). The patient must keep the distal thumb joint extended. Early weakness is indicated if the patient is forced to flex the thumb to resist the examiner. As an alternate technique, the patient can resist the examiner's attempt to pull a card from the grip of the adducted thumb (distal joint extended) against the first finger, or the patient can grasp both ends of the paper in this manner and resist the examiner's attempt to pull his hands apart. The weaker muscle will let go first.

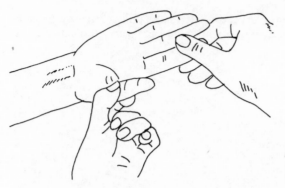

Fig. 3-24. Adductor pollicis. The examiner attempts to pull away the thumb.

Interossei—Ulnar Nerve, C8-T1 The dorsal and palmar interossei and the lumbricales are involved, along with extensors and flexors, in skilled movements of the hand. The interossei and lumbricales have two sources of innervation (ulnar and median nerves) that can be variable. The examiner interlocks his fingers with the patient's and resists the patient's attempts to adduct (Fig. 3-25) and abduct (Fig. 3-26) his fingers. The patient is instructed not to use his thumb.

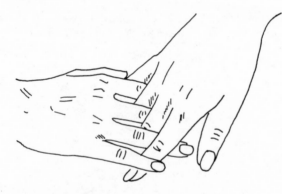

Fig. 3-25. Interossei. The examiner attempts to separate the patient's tightly adducted fingers.

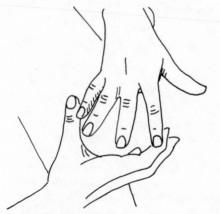

Fig. 3-26. Interossei. The examiner attempts to adduct the patient's tightly abducted fingers.

Grip—Median and Ulnar Nerves, C8-T1 In testing the grip, various forms of dynamometers can be used by the examiner to obtain an objective measurement to compare both hands or to monitor change over a period of time. Such measurement by a dynamometer is often an effective way of differentiating malingering from true paralysis. It is hard for the malingerer to maintain a constant weakness at differing times. If there are other muscles weak in the forearm, the wrist must be supported for an effective grip. Both grips can be compared if the examiner attempts to pull his fingers out from the grip of both hands simultaneously.

Diaphragm—Phrenic Nerve, C3-C5 With tangential lighting, a shadow can be seen descending along the rib cage on inspiration. This is produced by the diaphragm as it peels off the inner chest wall. Action of the diaphragm in concert with the intercostals can be assayed by watching respiratory movements that include flaring of the ribs and the elevation of the epigastrium.

Intercostals—Intercostal Nerves, T1-T12 Palpation of the intercostal muscles with fingertips between the ribs can offer information about their contractile strength. Resistance applied by the examiner's hands to the expanding chest wall during inspiration can challenge intercostal strength. Careful observation of the chest wall and its symmetry of movement may reveal unilateral lag or decreased amplitude indicating poor intercostal strength, guarding due to pain, or poor aeration of one lung.

> Although variations occur in the predominance of chest or intercostal muscle action over abdominal or diaphragmatic muscle action in normal respiration, both sets of muscles should move in synchrony. Seesaw, opposite, or paradoxical movements might indicate diaphragmatic weakness. The use of accessory muscles indicate respiratory embarrassment due either to weakness of the respiratory muscles or a blocked airway. In the comatose patient, obstruction can be caused by a slack jaw or unswallowed secretion in the pharynx.

Respiration A very rough estimate of the patient's ventilatory capacity can be made by watching the patient count rapidly in sequence as far as possible on one breath after maximum inspiration. Normally, the adult patient can get to around 40 before another breath is necessary.

> Although there is a large degree of individual variation in the test, it does allow for subsequent evaluation to determine whether there is a change in the patient's respiratory capacity. This must be regarded as a very crude but convenient test. Whenever ventilatory insufficiency is possible or suspected, more accurate measurement should be made with a ventilometer. Unilateral or bilateral diaphragmatic paresis can be seen on radiographic fluoroscopy.

Abdominals—T5-L1 The examiner observes the patient's abdominal muscle strength and palpates the contracting muscles as the patient elevates his head from the table or attempts to sit without using the arms (ask him to cross his arms on his chest).

> If the lower abdominal muscles are weak due to a lesion at the level of T8, the umbilicus will move toward the head as the patient sits up. This elevation is caused

by the unopposed pull of the intact upper abdominal muscles. This is a helpful observation in determining the level of motor paralysis in a patient who has paraplegia. In the normal person, no displacement of the umbilicus occurs on contraction of the abdominal muscles.

Leg Extensors: Quadriceps and Ilipsoas—Femoral Nerve, L2-L4 Pressing down on the extended leg near the ankle, the examiner tests the combined iliopsoas and quadriceps (Fig. 3-27).

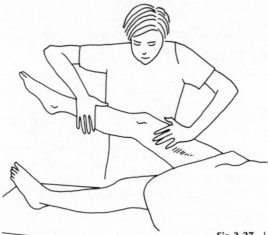

Fig. 3-27. Leg extensors: quadriceps and iliopsoas

Iliopsoas—Femoral Nerve, L1-L3 Action of the iliopsoas is isolated by flexing the knee and asking the patient to move his knee toward his chest against resistance applied by the examiner at the knee (Fig. 3-28).

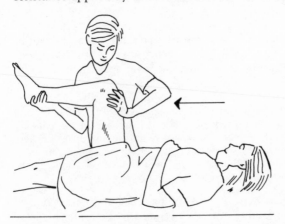

Fig. 3-28. Iliopsoas. The examiner resists the patient's attempt to flex her knee to her chest.

Quadriceps—Femoral Nerve, L2-L4 The patient extends the knee against the examiner's resistance at the ankle (Fig. 3-29). The more the patient's knee is flexed at the outset, the easier the quadriceps will be overcome by the examiner. Note the support given to the leg under the knee by the examiner.

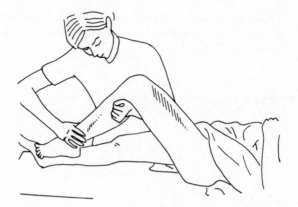

Fig. 3-29. Quadriceps

Hamstrings—Sciatic Nerve, L4-S2 The patient flexes the knee against the examiner's resistance at the ankle (Fig. 3-30). This muscle can seem surprisingly weak in comparison to the antigravity quadriceps muscle.

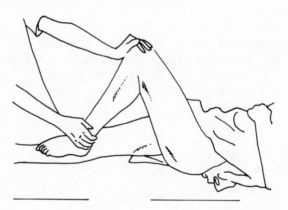

Fig. 3-30. Hamstrings. Tendons and contracting muscles can be seen.

Adductors of the Thigh—Obturator Nerve L2-L4 The examiner attempts to separate patient's legs against the patient's resistance (Fig. 3-31).

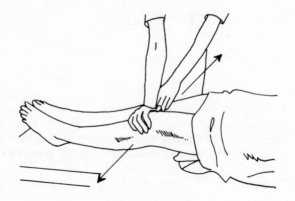

Fig. 3-31. Adductors of the thigh.

Abductors of the Thigh—Superior Gluteal Nerve, L4-S1 Here the patient attempts to abduct the thighs, or separate the knees against the examiner's resistance (Fig. 3-32).

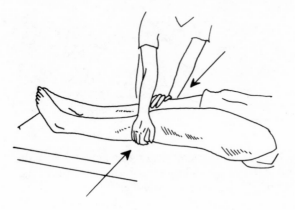

Fig. 3-32. Abductors of the thigh

Gastrocnemius—Sciatic Nerve, S1-S2 It is important to remember that this muscle, being an antigravity muscle, is almost impossible to adequately test with the patient lying in bed. The patient attempts to plantar flex the ankle against the examiner's resistance (Fig. 3-33). The better test is toe walking if the patient is ambulatory.

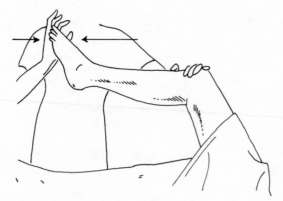

Fig. 3-33. Gastrocnemius. Note muscle belly contraction and tendon.

Dorsiflexors of the Foot—Deep Peroneal Nerve, L4-S1 This is an important muscle in all examination routines because of its early involvement in pyramidal hemiplegia or upper motor neuron deficits. The patient attempts to maintain dorsiflexion of the foot against the counterpressure of the examiner (Fig. 3-34).

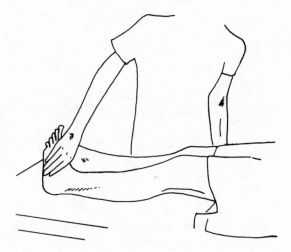

Fig. 3-34. Dorsiflexors of the foot

Extensor Hallucis Longus—Deep Peroneal Nerve, L5-S1 The patient dorsiflexes the great toe against counterpressure (Fig. 3-35). This is an excellent test for the L5 root.

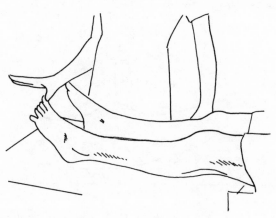

Fig. 3-35. Extensor hallucis longus

Peronei—Superficial Peroneal Nerve, L5-S1 The examiner inverts the foot and asks the patient to actively oppose this action (Fig. 3-36). Note the contracting tendons.

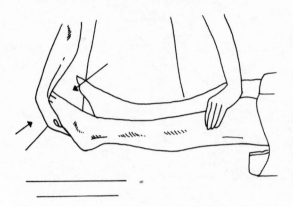

Fig. 3-36. Peronei. Tendons can be seen, as well as contraction of the small belly of the extensor digitorum brevis on the lateral dorsum of the foot. The patient everts the foot against the examiner's resistance.

Gluteus Maximus—Inferior Gluteal Nerve, L5-S2 The prone patient elevates a flexed knee against resistance of the examiner (Fig. 3-37). The muscle can be seen and palpated. Remember the gluteal test on the standing patient described previously as a better challenge to the gluteus medius. These are very strong muscles and weakness may be hard to detect.

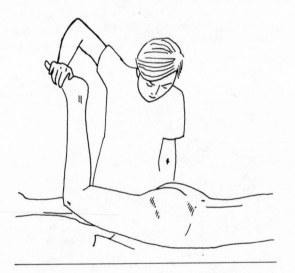

Fig. 3-37. Gluteus maximus

Extensors of the Back—C1-L5 The prone patient hyperextends the back by elevating the head off the bed without using his arms. The examiner can resist the action.

BACKGROUND DATA FOR MOTOR SYSTEM EXAMINATION

Involvement of the Upper Motor Neuron (Corticospinal or Pyramidal) System This can occur with lesions in the motor cortex, corona radiata, internal capsule, the "pyramidal" or corticospinal tract in the brain stem, and lateral columns of the spinal cord. This motor system is primarily involved in voluntary motor skills (Fig. 3-38).

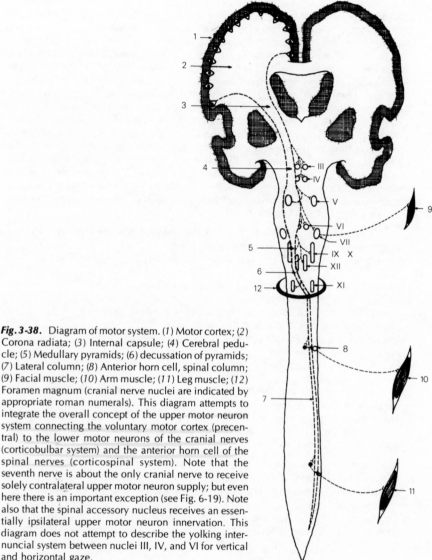

Fig. 3-38. Diagram of motor system. (*1*) Motor cortex; (*2*) Corona radiata; (*3*) Internal capsule; (*4*) Cerebral peduncle; (*5*) Medullary pyramids; (*6*) decussation of pyramids; (*7*) Lateral column; (*8*) Anterior horn cell, spinal column; (*9*) Facial muscle; (*10*) Arm muscle; (*11*) Leg muscle; (*12*) Foramen magnum (cranial nerve nuclei are indicated by appropriate roman numerals). This diagram attempts to integrate the overall concept of the upper motor neuron system connecting the voluntary motor cortex (precentral) to the lower motor neurons of the cranial nerves (corticobulbar system) and the anterior horn cell of the spinal nerves (corticospinal system). Note that the seventh nerve is about the only cranial nerve to receive solely contralateral upper motor neuron supply; but even here there is an important exception (see Fig. 6-19). Note also that the spinal accessory nucleus receives an essentially ipsilateral upper motor neuron innervation. This diagram does not attempt to describe the yolking internuncial system between nuclei III, IV, and VI for vertical and horizontal gaze.

The upper motor neuron, originating in the motor cortex, synapses with the lower motor neuron in the motor nuclei of the brain stem (corticobulbar system) or with the anterior horn cells of the spinal cord (corticospinal system). This lower motor neuron, in turn, synapses with muscles at their myoneural junction to produce muscle contraction. Paralysis, due to involvement of the upper motor neuron system, would be contralateral to the neural damage above the decussation of the pyramids (brain stem or cerebral hemisphere) and ipsilateral to damage in the lateral columns of the spinal cord. The pattern of weakness seen in the upper neuron involvement is characteristically that of a hemiplegia involving the arm and leg on the same side of the body; if the lesion is above the pons, the face is also involved. The degree of paralysis, and the degree of spasticity characteristic of upper motor neuron lesions can vary depending on the location and extent of the lesion. It is very important for the examiner to note the pattern of weakness, spasticity, alteration in the reflexes, and sensation, to make a decision about localization. With upper motor neuron lesions, the involved extremities are usually diffusely involved, except that the antigravity muscles tend to be less involved in the weakness pattern. This produces the characteristic early weakness of the dorsiflexors of the wrist and foot in hemiplegias. If a lesion in the brain stem or spinal cord involves the corticospinal systems bilaterally, the patient shows quadriparesis or paraparesis depending upon the level of the spinal cord or brain stem involvement. Although paraparesis of spinal cord origin shows considerable extensor spasticity, it may present as flexor spasticity. It is possible for a monoplegia to occur in the leg with involvement of the lateral column below the segments innervating the arm, or as the result of discrete lesions in the motor cortex. Occasionally, a spastic paraparesis can be seen with sagittal lesions of the cerebrum (usually meningiomas) that impinge on the medial motor cortex bilaterally (leg area). Listed below are the characteristics that distinguish upper motor neuron involvement from other types of weakness.

Characteristics of Involvement of the Upper Motor Neuron System

Weakness without early or exceptional atrophy

Hyperactive stretch reflexes and often clonus (usually ankle and occasionally patellar)

Extensor plantar reflex or other pathological reflexes in the foot *Babinski*

Increased tone or spasticity

Clumsy performance in skilled movements with hands or feet

Dragging of the ball of the foot during walking

Circumducting movements of the hip during walking *→ to compensate*

Flexed posture of the arm

Externally rotated extended leg when supine

Reduced arm swing on walking

Arm pronation downward drift and elbow flexion on prolonged extension of the arm with palms upward

Trunk-thigh sign on sitting up from a supine position; higher than normal elevation of the paretic leg during the sitting up process

Reduced pendulousness

With minimal involvement, only extensor plantar reflex, minimal dorsiflexor weakness, and clumsiness may be seen. The experienced examiner may feel that upper motor neuron weakness is present even without any one of these minimal signs on examination.

Corticospinal involvement may be present without hypertonia, spasticity, or even hyperactive deep tendon reflexes in certain instances. This may be caused by "spinal

---

Fig. 3-39. Diagram of cerebellar system. (*1*) Motor cortex; (*2*) Pontine nuclei; (*3*) Middle cerebral peduncle (brachium pontis); (*4*) Purkinje cell (neocerebellum) lateral lobes; (*5*) Deep cerebellar nuclei; (*6*) Superior cerebellar peduncle; (*7*) Red nucleus; (*8*) Thalamus; (*9*) Dorsal root ganglion with neuron bodies of sensory afferents from muscle spindle; (*10*) Dorsal and ventral spinocerebellar tracts; (*11*) Inferior cerebellar peduncle (restiform body); (*12*) Purkinje cell neuron, anterior lobe (paleocerebellum); (*13*) Reticular formation, neurons to reticulospinal pathway; (*14*) Vestibular nuclei; (*15*) Flocculonodular complex (archicerebellum); (*16*) Inferior olive; (*17*) Anterior horn cell (lower motor neuron); (*18*) Skeletal muscle. (The dotted vertical line represents the midline.) This diagram demonstrates the connections to the cerebellum and its "feedback loop" connections to the motor system at cerebral cortical (neocerebellum), spinal (paleocerebellum) and vestibular (archicerebellum) levels.

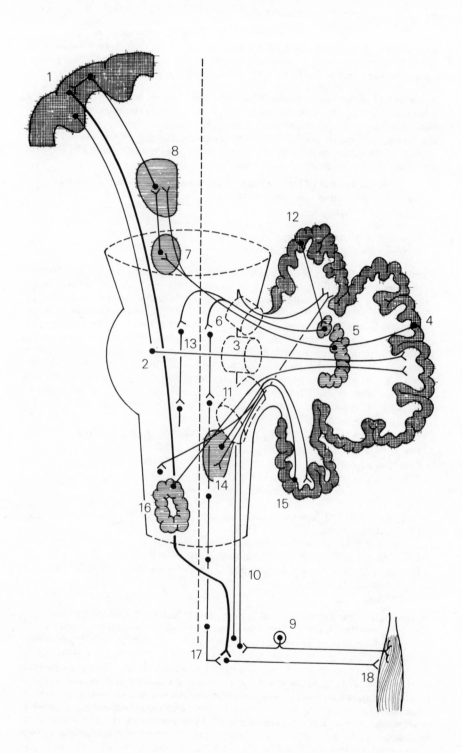

shock" seen in patients with acute spinal cord lesions, acute cerebral lesions, and small focal motor cortex lesions. The former two conditions eventually do show spasticity and increased reflexes after a variable length of time.

Involvement of the Lower Motor Neuron System This includes lesions of anterior horn cell, the motor root, the peripheral nerve, or its terminal endings in muscle. The pattern of muscle involvement or weakness depends upon the anatomic location of the lesion (*i.e.*, spinal cord, motor root, plexus, peripheral nerve) as well as the multiplicity, focality, or diffuseness of the lesion. Lower motor neuron involvement has many of the following characteristics on examination.

Characteristics of Involvement of the Lower Motor Neuron System
Weakness associated with early muscle atrophy
Hypotonia or flaccidity
Fasciculation (with anterior horn or root involvement)
Reduced or absent deep tendon reflexes
Trophic changes of the skin and nail bed

Involvement of the Cerebellar Systems Cerebellar symptoms and signs can be seen with lesions of either the cerebellum, the sensory pathways to the cerebellum, or the efferent motor pathways to the cerebral hemisphere from the cerebellum (Fig. 3-39). Cerebellar involvement characteristically shows clinical signs and symptoms ipsilateral to the cerebellar lesions. Cerebellar symptomatology can clear rapidly with nonprogressive focal hemisphere lesions of the cerebellum. It is important for the examiner to remember that cerebellar signs can be due to inadequate proprioceptive sensory information, conscious or unconscious, reaching the cerebellum via the spinal cord from muscle spindles and joint receptors. Midline or vermal lesions involve balance or equilibrium with the trunk and legs. Lateral or hemispheric lesions usually involve extremity coordination. The phenomena listed below may be seen in patients with cerebellar involvement.

Characteristics of Involvement of the Cerebellar Systems
Finger-to-nose, heel-to-toe dysmetria
Intention tremor
Ataxia of gait, in extremity or trunk
Lack of check (or rebound phenomenon)
Pendulousness
"Macrographic handwriting" (wide ranging, rising circular script)
Dysdiadochokinesis
Outward drift of the arm on extension with eyes closed
Broad-based gait (difficulty with normal, narrow-based gait)
Decomposition of movement (absence of smooth sequence of muscle activity in coordinated limb movements)
Dysarthria

Involvement of the Extrapyramidal System (Basal Nuclei or Ganglia) This produces symptoms and signs contralateral to the lesion (Fig. 3-40). The symptoms and signs of extrapyramidal disease disappear in sleep and can be remarkably minimized during relaxation. However, the symptoms and signs can be remarkably intensified by examination, anxiety, tension, and illness. It seems apparent that the extrapyramidal system deals with postural muscle tone, automatic stereotyped or unconscious repetitive movements, and maintenance of normal reciprocal muscle tone as in postural maintenance. The extrapyramidal system undoubtedly involves not only the basal nuclei (or ganglia) and various nuclei of the brain stem, but also areas in the motor cortex. The exact anatomical limits of the functioning extrapyramidal system in the nervous system is debatable. The following varieties of the symptoms and signs can be seen with disease of the extrapyramidal system.

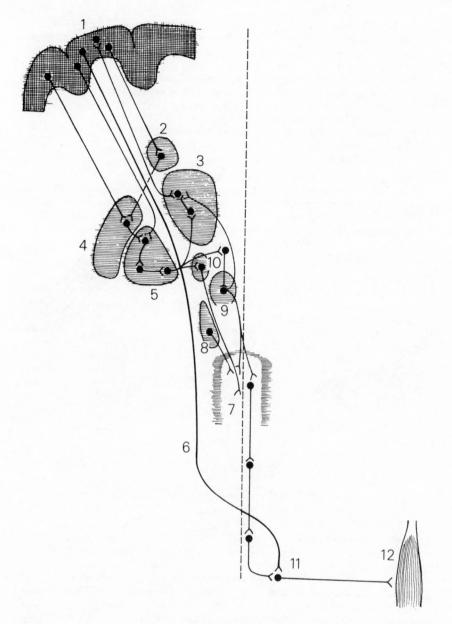

Fig. 3-40. Diagram of the extrapyramidal system. (*1*) motor cortex; (*2*) Caudate nucleus; (*3*) Thalamus; (*4*) Putamen; (*5*) Globus pallidus; (*6*) Corticospinal tract; (*7*) Reticular formation; (*8*) Substantia nigra; (*9*) Red nucleus; (*10*) Subthalamic nucleus; (*11*) Anterior horn cell (lower motor neuron); (*12*) Skeletal muscle. This diagram only sketchily shows the rich interconnections of the basal nuclei involved in the "extrapyramidal system." Note that this system, intimately interconnected with the corticospinal, corticobulbar, and cerebellar systems, can affect the anterior horn cell (lower motor neuron) either by connections with the motor cortex or by descending connections through the reticulospinal and rubrospinal systems. The globus pallidus is the principal outflow of this integrated system.

Characteristics of Involvement of the Extrapyramidal System

Tremor (postural, often but not always diminished on intention)

Akinesia or paucity of spontaneous movement with disinclination or effort in initiating movement

Hyperkinesias: Chorea, athetosis, dystonia, and ballism

Rigidity: Cogwheel (superimposed tremor); plastic (resistance unchanging at all degrees of extension and flexion; shortening and lengthening of the tendons in maintaining constant resistance or "tone")

"Micrographic writing" (small, jagged, falling, tight script)

Postural abnormalities

Loss of facial expression

Diffuse Symmetrical Weakness It is important for the examiner to differentiate at the side of the patient, if at all possible, the probable anatomical site involved in patients who have diffuse, symmetrical, bilateral weakness. Such weakness can be due to involvement in many different places of the neuromuscular unit. The following clinical anatomic correlation may prove helpful in such evaluation (see Fig. 3-41).

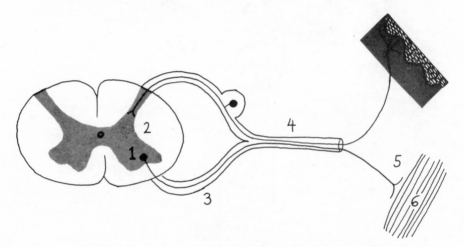

Fig. 3-41. Diagram of the neuromuscular unit (See text for description.)

1. Anterior horn cell involvement, as seen in the progressive motor neuron diseases, evidences flaccidity, atrophy, early fasciculations, and often a distal distribution of muscle weakness. There is no sensory involvement.
2. In diffuse involvement of a spinal cord segment, there is often evidence of lower motor neuron weakness at the level of the cord lesion and signs of upper motor neuron weakness below the cord lesion due to corticospinal tract involvement. There is also evidence of sensory loss in a dermatomal pattern at the level of the lesion and for an indefinite number of segments below (see the discussion of sensory examination on p. 59).
3. Multiple root involvement as radiculitis seen in patients with the Guillain-Barré syndrome shows segmental motor paralysis in a root distribution, primarily of distal muscles, and a dermatomal sensory loss. There may be muscle spasm and radiating pain in some cases. Most impressive in this type of lesion is the diffuse loss of stretch reflexes. Lesions of longer duration eventually show atrophy primarily in a distal distribution and patchy fasciculations.

4. Muscle weakness due to diffuse peripheral nerve disease as in polyneuritis or polyneuropathy often shows a "stocking-glove" sensory loss and a primarily distal motor weakness, with atrophy and loss of reflexes of the lower motor neuron type. Autonomic changes in skin texture, loss of hair, changes in the nail beds, changes in temperature, and color changes in the limb can be seen.

5. Involvement of the myoneural junction, as seen in myasthenia gravis, may show diffuse muscle weakness usually without evidence of atrophy or reflex alteration. There is a characteristic aggravation of the weakness by continued effort and improvement with rest. No sensory losses are seen.

6. Diffuse weakness due to muscle involvement (e.g., myopathy, dystrophy, polymyositis) shows symmetric muscle weakness involving primarily proximal muscles of the shoulder girdle and/or pelvic girdle. There may or may not be atrophy. (There can be pseudohypertrophy in some forms of dystrophy.) There may or may not be tenderness, contracture of the muscles, and normal muscle irritability. There is usually minimal alteration in the reflexes. Electromyography, serum enzymes studies, and muscle biopsy may be very helpful in the analysis of these problems.

4

THE SENSORY SYSTEM

Evaluation of the sensory system is the least objective portion of the neurologic examination since the examiner must depend completely upon the patient's report of what he feels. The reliability of the patient's report varies with his suggestibility, fatigue, attitude concerning the illness, rapport with the examiner, ability to communicate, and sensitivity to stimuli.

Absent sensation is obvious when it is found, but the examiner should seek any variation in sensation from what he would normally expect from the stimulus he is using. Variations in both quality and degree of sensation must be sought. The following definitions, although not universally recognized, will be useful.

Analgesia—absence of pain or pin sensation
Anesthesia—absence of sensation, usually to touch
Hypesthesia—reduced touch sensation
Hypalgesia—decreased pain or pin sensation
Hyperesthesia—increased sensation, usually to touch
Dysesthesia—bizarre sensation or sensations elicited by a stimulus
Paresthesia—spontaneously occurring abnormal sensations, such as "pins and needles"
Hyperpathia—exaggerated pain response, usually to a stimulus

Avoid tiring the patient with the sensory examination, or he may give inaccurate answers. This examination may need to be deferred until the patient is refreshed. The patient's eyes should be closed during most of the sensory examination. Explain carefully what you are doing to the patient and demand clear-cut answers. Reliability can be checked by repeating the sensory examination some hours later. A skin-marking pencil can be used to delineate topography of altered sensation on the patient's body.

EXTEROCEPTIVE SENSATION

This refers to the reception of stimuli from the surface of the skin; it is tested through the modalities of pin stimulation (or "pain"), temperature, and light touch. Exteroceptive pathways seem relatively well defined in the central nervous system (spinothalamic and quintothalamic pathways).

Pin Testing

This procedure should not be uncomfortable to the average patient if the examiner uses a light tap or scratch with a loosely held pin drawn at an acute angle.

It is impossible, and uncomfortable for the patient, to survey the entire body with the pin; the examiner attempts to sample areas characteristically affected by neurological lesions involving peripheral nerves or dermatomes. To avoid fatiguing the patient, and to assist him in making decisions, the examiner should make the following comparisons.

1. Compare the face to the hand and leg.
2. Compare left and right sides of the face, trunk, arms and legs.
3. Compare distal to proximal sensations by sequential pin stimulations up the extremities.
4. Compare medial, lateral, anterior, and posterior aspects of the extremities by circumferential pin testing (note dermatomal and peripheral nerve sensory charts).

Be sure to ask the patient if the stimuli "feel the same" or "equal." If you ask a suggestible patient, "Is there a difference?," you may focus attention on differences that are not of consequence. Be certain to ask the patient what the stimulus feels like; just admitting he feels it is no assurance that it feels sharp. If there is evidence of sensory alteration, then the examiner must search more thoroughly and assiduously for the actual pattern of the sensory loss to determine if it suggests peripheral nerve, sensory root, plexus, polyneuropathy, or central nervous system involvement (see p. 59).

To map out sensory losses, always start with the least sensitive area and travel to the area of greater sensation for accurate demarcation. This means from hypesthetic to normal, or from normal to hyperesthetic. Use a skin pencil and recheck frequently. The results of sensory examination should be drawn on a body map on the patient's chart.

Recognition of a Sharp Stimulus With the eyes closed, the patient is asked whether he feels a sharp or dull sensation as the examiner randomly alternates sharp and dull stimuli over various parts of the body. This maneuver is helpful in verifying sensory loss on pin stimulation in patients in whom reliability is a question or cooperation is difficult. Tricking the patient may be necessary in verifying the accuracy of his report.

Sequential Pin Testing Unless the examiner goes sequentially from toe to head with a repetitive pin stimulus on both sides of the body, he may miss a dermatomal sensory loss. This is especially true in thoracic and abdominal root lesions and in cord lesions producing isolated zones of hypesthesia. "Peek-a-boo" pin testing in and around clothing is fraught with disaster. The pin may feel sharp on the legs and on the arms, but both you and the patient might be surprised if a sequentially moving pin discovered a sudden increase or decrease in sensation over the trunk.

Temperature Testing A container of truly hot water and a container of crushed ice should be used. Unless the stimuli are clearly cold and hot on immediate contact with the skin, the results can be confusing. Test tubes or metal syringe containers are convenient. Since moisture may condense on the cold container, it should be dried to prevent identification by moisture alone. The examiner should avoid applying alternate stimuli in sequence on the same spot of the body. Again, the patient must be adequately disrobed and thoroughly tested. Temperature testing is not routinely performed unless there is sensory loss elicited on the examination with a pin, the patient gives the history of sensory changes, or a neurological problem exists that suggests a temperature sensation may be important in the total assessment of the problem. For a quick check, a cold instrument can be used (until it warms by repeated body contact).

Light Touch

The patient is asked to identify when he is touched by the lightest whisk of cotton with the eyes closed. This modality is usually used to confirm previously elicited sensory loss on pin stimulation (as in peripheral nerve disorders) or to discover dissociation of pin and touch (pin and/or temperature sensation decreased, touch intact) as seen in patients with intramedullary spinal cord lesions.

Some examiners prefer to use this stimulus in the place of pin testing for the sake of comfort. However, quantitative changes are less likely to be noticed by the patient, and valuable data could be overlooked. Touch travels more diffusely in the nervous system and by many different routes (*e.g.,* spinothalamic, posterior column).

On body surfaces, the distribution of touch fibers may overlap considerably so that more than one peripheral nerve may have to be involved before loss of sensation is detected.

PROPRIOCEPTIVE SENSATION

This refers to the conscious reception of stimuli from joints, joint capsules, tendons, and deep receptors in the skin and muscle tissue; it is information from within the body (posterior columns–medial lemniscus). Neurophysiological studies suggest that sensory information from annulospiral muscle endings on intrafusal muscle fibers and Golgi-tendon organs goes to the cerebellum, brain stem, and local cord segments, and is not consciously received at cortical levels. This information provides the central nervous system and the motor system with information concerning the length, tension, and movement of the skeletal muscles used for integrated motor performance (spinocerebellar pathways).

Romberg Test

In this examination, the patient is asked to stand with feet together and eyes closed. The patient must be able to stand steadily with eyes open before a comparison with the eyes closed can be made. The ability to stand with eyes closed depends upon the integrity of the proprioceptive information from the sensory endings in the foot ascending up the posterior columns. The Romberg test should be thought of as a test of posterior column function; it is not a cerebellar test per se. The test is positive if the patient sways markedly or cannot stand with the eyes closed. The play of tendons on the dorsum of the foot while the patient is standing with the eyes closed indicates rapid compensatory motor movements reflexly sent down the cord as a result of intact unconscious proprioception ascending the cord to brain stem and cerebellar levels (spinocerebellar tract). A positive Romberg test usually indicates a posterior column disorder. Patients with cerebellar disease have difficulty standing with eyes open; this might be exaggerated slightly when the eyes are closed.

Vibration Sensation

This test should be performed with the patient's eyes closed. The tuning fork should have a frequency of 128 cps and produce a strong vibration that decreases slowly. The tuning fork is applied repeatedly up the body, distal to proximal, until its vibration is perceived. The examiner can check for diminished sensation by comparing the patient's response to his own. Good reception in the toes or ankles usually precludes further testing unless the examiner feels that the patient has cervical, thoracic root, or spinal cord disease. Although the tuning fork is traditionally applied to bony prominences, there is no rationale for this other than the possible convenience of a bony prominence for contact by the fork to the patient's body. The tuning fork can be applied directly to the skin or with the examiner's finger between the tuning fork and the patient's body. It is important to be sure that the patient feels vibration as a sensation when the tuning fork is applied ("buzzing" or "humming"), not just a touch sensation.

Responses to vibration stimuli are notoriously unreliable even in cooperative patients. In order to check the accuracy of the patient's responses, it is often valuable for the examiner to apply (without the patient's knowledge) a nonvibrating tuning fork to areas of the body where the patient claims he perceives vibration.

> Vibration sensation is perceived consciously at the thalamic level in the contralateral hemisphere. This sensation is intact in patients with parietal cortex damage and lost in those with thalamic damage. With many varieties of spinal cord lesions, vibration sensation may be lost although position sense is still intact. Vibration sensibility is often diminished in the feet in older patients. There is some evidence that vibration sensation may travel in pathways other than the posterior columns. Clinically, it is useful to consider it as mediated by the posterior columns.

Position Sensation

The patient's eyes should be closed for this examination. The examiner bends, or extends, the great toe or other toe and asks the patient in which way the toe was moved (Fig. 4-1). Position sense in the fingers is tested in the same manner. The examiner should be careful that only the joint examined is moved (Fig. 4-2). If the patient cannot detect movement in the peripheral part of the extremity, as the toes or the fingers, or cannot indicate the direction they are pointing, then the ankles, wrists, knees, and elbows should be similarly tested to determine the level of position sense loss.

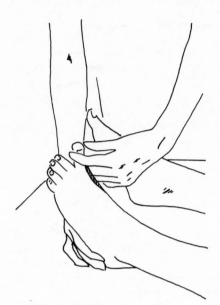

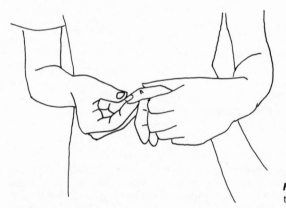

Fig. 4-1. Position sense testing in the great toe

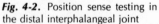

Fig. 4-2. Position sense testing in the distal interphalangeal joint

Position and vibration tests do not duplicate each other, and both should be tested.

There is another method of showing loss of position sensation, especially in the upper extremity. The patient, with eyes closed, holds the affected arm in an unusual position, then tries to point with his other hand to the location of the postured hand, or to mimic the same posture with his other extremities.

Deep Pain Sensation

Deep pain sensory pathways can be tested by squeezing the Achilles tendon or testicles, forcibly flexing the digits, or pinching the belly of the pectoralis muscle anterior to the axilla. Deep pain sensation travels by proprioceptive pathways and is notably lost or diminished in patients with diseases of the posterior roots (*e.g.,* tabes dorsalis).

DISCRIMINATIVE SENSATION *(cortical function (is parietal)*

This refers to sensory decisions requiring perception and integration of sensory information at the level of the parietal cortex. Sensory pathways, especially proprioception, must be intact. Position sense, for example, is not only a test of proprioceptive pathways, but also a test of parietal cortex integrity since the cortical decision "up" or "down" must be made in response to the information received. Stereognosis, graphesthesia, and two-point sensation are aspects of discriminative or cortical function.

Stereognosis

With eyes closed, the patient is asked to identify an object by its feel, shape, texture, and weight. The examiner should see that the patient does not transfer the object to another hand, and should be sure the patient receives no auditory information about the object (*e.g.,* click of a comb or tinkle of keys). Intactness of proprioception can be assumed, even before the patient answers, by the intelligent or knowing way he feels the object.

Graphesthesia

The patient is asked to identify numbers drawn by the examiner on the palm or dorsum of the hand with a moderately sharp object. It can also be tested on the feet, arms, and legs. This is a useful test when paralysis prevents grasping of an object for the stereognosis testing.

Two-Point Sensation

Two similar pointed objects are used in this examination. The patient, with eyes closed, is instructed to say whether he is being touched by one or two points applied in random combination by the examiner. The examiner attempts to identify the maximum separation of two points in which the patient will still claim he is touched by one point. The sensitivity to two points varies with portions of the body. It is almost impossible to separate the two points more than a millimeter on the lips and the fingertips without their being identified as two points. As the examiner proceeds more proximally and more dorsally, the distance required to identify two points becomes wider and wider. On the back, the examiner may frequently have stimuli several centimeters apart, and the patient still feels as though he is touched by one point. This examination is as important for sensory testing in peripheral nerve loss as it is in cortical sensory testing. Comparisons can only be made between the right and left sides.

Simultaneous Bilateral Sensation

With the patient's eyes closed, the examiner asks the patient to identify which extremity is touched and on which side. He then strokes or pricks the body on various homologous points unilaterally, and then bilaterally, simultaneously to see if the patient recognizes the bilateral stimuli.

With involvement of the parietal lobe or the thalamoparietal radiations, there may be no loss of touch or pin sensation when the pin is applied unilaterally. However, loss of sensory perception on the contralateral side of the body may be elicited if stimuli are applied to both sides of the body simultaneously. This phenomenon has been variously called inattention, or suppression, of bilateral stimuli and is related to delayed sensory "processing" by the involved parietal cortex. The phenomenon can also be seen in the visual fields as described in the section on cranial nerve examination (see p. 93). This test is a subtle challenge for discriminative sensory function by the parietal lobe in the bedside examination.

SIGNS OF PARIETAL LOBE LESIONS

Parietal lobe lesions may produce loss of primary sensations for discriminative sensations on the opposite side of the body. Cortical sensory loss, due to acute anterior parietal lobe lesions, can be global, initially involving sensitivity to pin prick and touch. In more chronic or slowly developing lesions, parietal cortex damage is usually characterized by

Loss of position sense
Loss of discriminative sensation
Preservation of tactile, temperature, and pain sensations (these can be affected)
Preservation of vibration sensation

More posteriorly located lesions in the parietal cortex produce astereognosia and many other "parietal lobe phenomena." It is important to understand the different constellations of symptoms and signs that can occur if the parietal lobe lesions are in the right or left parietal cortex. Left and right designations below refer to the usual right-handed patient and also to left-handed patients who have their language skills in the left cerebral cortex.

Possible Signs of Right Parietal Lesions

Astereognosis on the left side
Inattention to bilateral simultaneous stimuli on the left
Patient's lack of recognition of left side, arm, and/or leg (autotopagnosia)
Left-sided body neglect on dressing, grooming, or arranging bed clothing. (The patient acts as if totally unaware of the left side of the body.)
Unawareness or lack of ability to identify left-sided defect as paralysis (anosognosia)
Left-sided disorientation
Spatial disorientation (e.g., in interpretation of compass directions, map reading, spatial relationships, three dimensional figures)
Left-sided tactile stimuli felt on homologous areas of the right side or incorrectly located on the left
Kinesthetic illusions of movement in limbs on left side

Possible Signs of Left Parietal Lesions

Spatial disorientation (e.g., in interpretation of compass directions, map reading)
On bilateral stimulation, inattention to stimuli from the right
Astereognosis, graphesthesia, loss of position sense, and two-point discrimination all on the right side
Visual agnosia in the interpretation of diagrams and maps (Popelreuter diagrams)
Constructional apraxia when the patient is asked to construct figures with matches or copy designs

Finger agnosia; inability to distinguish or name his own fingers or the examiner's
Right-left disorientation
Acalculia (poor mathematical skills)
Apraxia of the arm or leg
Various types of communication disorders (see Chapter 8)

It is important to remember that lesions of the parietal lobe, a so-called "silent" area of the brain, may produce no symptoms and signs.

SENSORY LOSS PATTERNS

The following illustrations should help the examiner delineate the pattern of sensory loss in his patient so that he can determine the extent of involvement and whether the sensory problems are of cortical, central, spinal, root, or peripheral nerve origins.

Dermatomal Sensory Patterns Two variations of the sensory areas on the skin served by the spinal cord segments or sensory roots are shown. Figure 4-3 (adapted from Haymaker and Woodhall, Peripheral Nerve Injuries, 2nd ed. W. B. Saunders, Philadelphia, 1953) is based on the body areas of intact sensation when roots above and below an isolated root were interrupted, sensation loss when one or more continuous roots were interrupted, or the pattern of herpetic rash and hypersensitivity in isolated root involvement. This schema shows areas smaller than actual root supply, as there is always considerable overlap in the body areas supplied by consecutive roots. These diagrams are most helpful in evaluating sensory loss in root or cord disease.

The dermatomal pattern shown in Figure 4-4 (adapted from Keegan, J. J. and Garrett, E. D. Anat. Record 102:4, pp. 409-439, 1943) is based on hyposensitivity to pin scratch in various root lesions, and is consistent with electrical skin resistance studies showing axial dermatomes extending to the distal extremities. This pattern is helpful in evaluating paresthesias and hypersthesias secondary to root irritation.

The examiner should be aware of both patterns in the evaluation of his patient. The heavy lines represent the ventral and dorsal axial lines about which the distal extension of the axial dermatomes rotate following the embryological growth of the extremities. This causes dermatomes not in sequential continuity to abut.

The Foerster dermatome map shows the "onion peel" pattern of facial sensory areas that relate to brain stem segments (as opposed to the trigeminal peripheral nerve pattern).

Peripheral Nerve Fields The diagrams shown in Figure 4-5 (adapted from Haymaker and Woodhall, Peripheral Nerve Injuries, 2nd Ed. W. B. Saunders, Philadelphia, 1953) indicate the skin areas that are provided sensory innervation by single peripheral nerves. Because of overlapping areas of innervation by peripheral nerves, these areas of isolated supply are smaller than the total area provided by a single peripheral nerve.

Contrast this pattern with the pattern of dermatomal areas seen clinically in sensory root or spinal cord involvement. Plexus lesions will, of course, produce different patterns; it is amazing how little sensory loss may be found in plexus lesions. The areas supplied by the posterior, lateral, and anterior rami of the thoracic or intercostal nerves are lumped together since they do not differ from the root or dermatomal pattern, as there is no intervening plexus.

(Text continues on page 67)

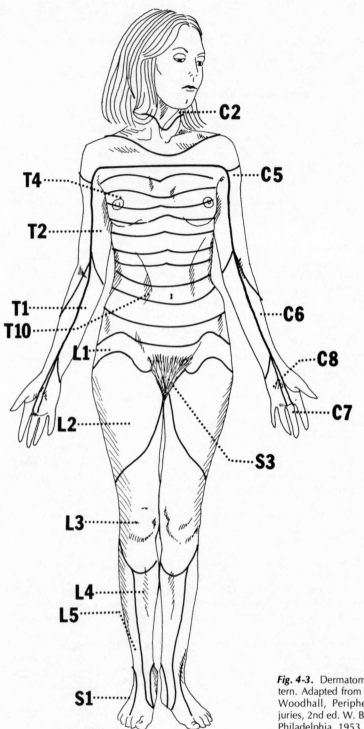

Fig. 4-3. Dermatomal sensory pattern. Adapted from Haymaker and Woodhall, Peripheral Nerve Injuries, 2nd ed. W. B. Saunders Co., Philadelphia, 1953.

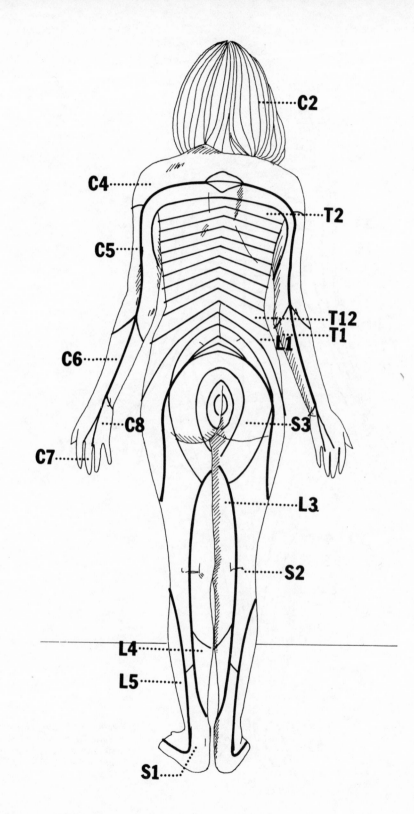

C2

C4

T2

C5

T12
T1
L1

C6

C8

S3

C7

L3

S2

L4

L5

S1

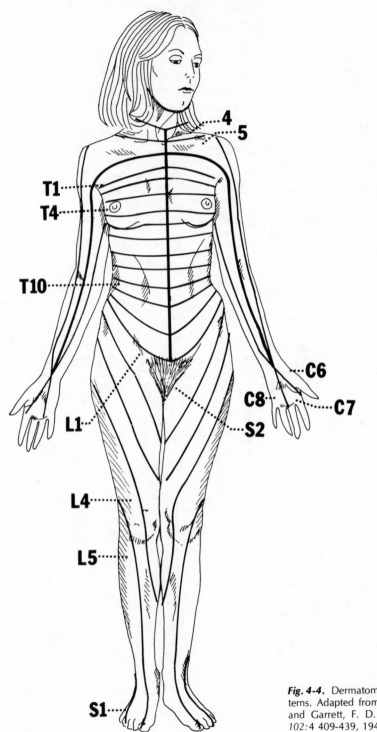

Fig. 4-4. Dermatomal sensory patterns. Adapted from Keegan, J. J., and Garrett, F. D. Anat. Record *102:*4 409-439, 1943.

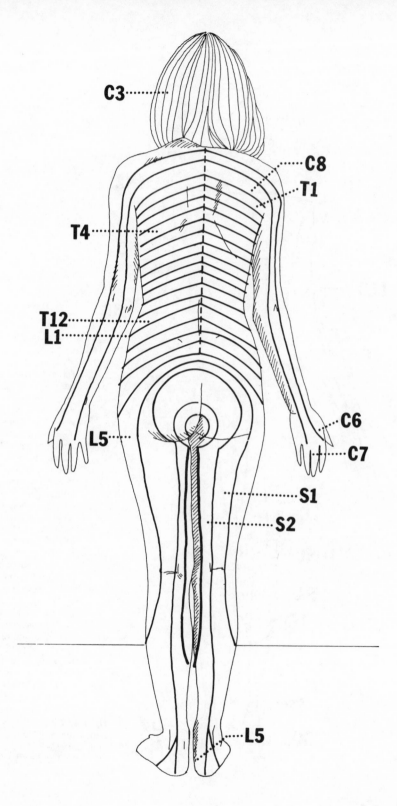

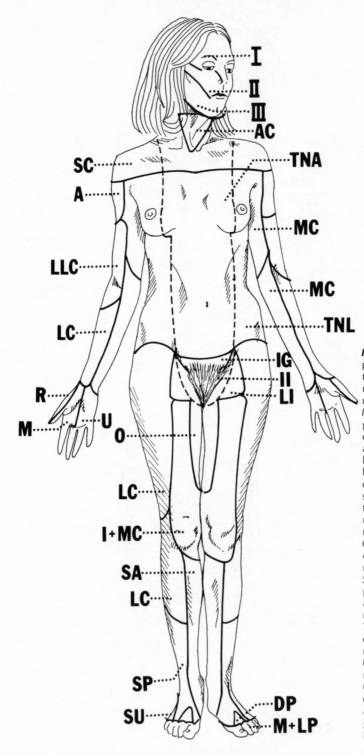

Fig. 4-5. Peripheral nerve sensory patterns. *A,* axillary nerve; *AC,* anterior cutaneous nerve; *CA,* calcanean branches of sural and tibial nerves; *DP,* deep peroneal nerve; *IG,* iliohypogastric nerve; *II,* illioinguinal nerve; *IMC,* inferior medial clunial nerve; *I+MC,* intermediate and medial cutaneous nerve; *LC,* lateral cutaneous nerve; *LI,* lumboinguinal nerve; *LLC,* lower lateral cutaneous nerve; *LS + CP,* lumbar, sacral and coccygeal nerves, posterior rami; *M,* median nerve; *MC,* medial cutaneous nerve; *M + LP,* medial and lateral plantar nerves; *O,* obturator nerve; *PC,* posterior cutaneous nerve, arm and thigh; *R,* radial nerve; *SA,* saphenous nerve; *SC,* supraclavicular nerve; *SP,* superficial peroneal nerve; *SU,* sural and plantar nerves; *TNA,* thoracic nerves, anterior cutaneous rami; *TNL,* thoracic nerves lateral cutaneous rami; *TNP,* thoracic nerves, posterior, cutaneous, rami; *U,* ulnar nerve; *I, II + III,* trigeminal nerve, peripheral diversions (ophthlamic, maxillary and mandibular). Adapted from Haymaker and Woodhall, Peripheral Nerve Injuries, 2nd Ed. W. B. Sanders Co. Philadelphia, 1953.

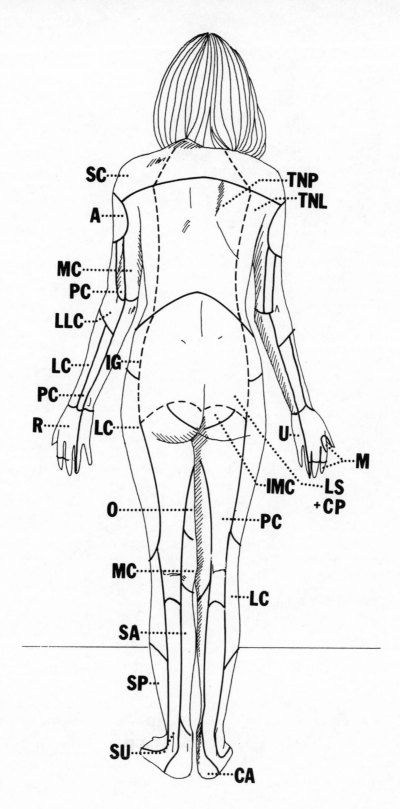

SC
TNP
TNL
A
MC
PC
LLC
LC
IG
PC
R
LC
U
M
IMC
LS
+CP
O
PC
MC
LC
SA
SP
SU
CA

65

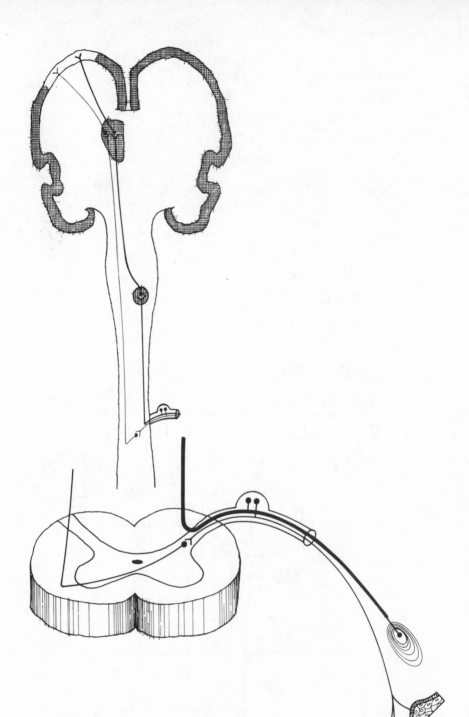

Fig. 4-6. Sensory pathways in the nervous system, for exteroceptive sensations: pin, temperature and light touch are indicated by the thin fibers. Proprioceptive sensations: position, vibration and touch are indicated by the thick fibers.

SENSORY PATHWAYS

Considerations of the conventionally described pathways for sensation will help to reinforce the localization value of sensory patterns (Fig. 4-6).

Pain (pin) and temperature or exteroceptive sensation mediated by slower conducting, poorly myelinated fibers makes a synaptic connection in the posterior horn of the spinal cord grey matter. The second order neuron crosses within a few segments, and its axon ascends to the thalamus (spinothalamic tract) where a third order neuron continues to the sensory (parietal) cortex. Proprioceptive sensation (vibration and position) utilizes more rapidly conducting fibers with thicker axons and heavier myelin sheaths. The axon of the first order neuron in the dorsal root ganglion, unlike the exteroceptive neuron, does not synapse at a cord segmented level but ascends uncrossed to the gracilis and cuneate nuclei in the caudal medulla. There the second order neuron crosses and ascends (medial lemniscus) to the thalamus joining the exteroceptive fibers in the spinothalamic tract. This difference in sensory pathways explains the patterns seen in Figure 4-7 *A* through *F*.

Fig. 4-7 *A* through *H* show the patterns in sensory deficit seen with lesions in various locations of the central and peripheral nervous system.

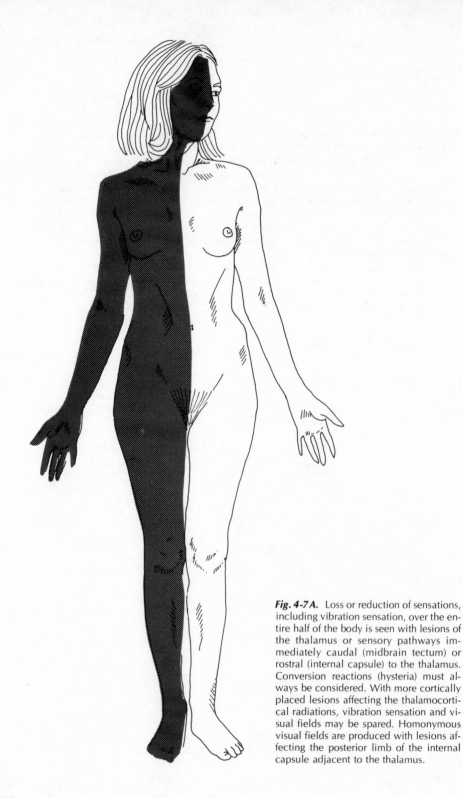

Fig. 4-7A. Loss or reduction of sensations, including vibration sensation, over the entire half of the body is seen with lesions of the thalamus or sensory pathways immediately caudal (midbrain tectum) or rostral (internal capsule) to the thalamus. Conversion reactions (hysteria) must always be considered. With more cortically placed lesions affecting the thalamocortical radiations, vibration sensation and visual fields may be spared. Homonymous visual fields are produced with lesions affecting the posterior limb of the internal capsule adjacent to the thalamus.

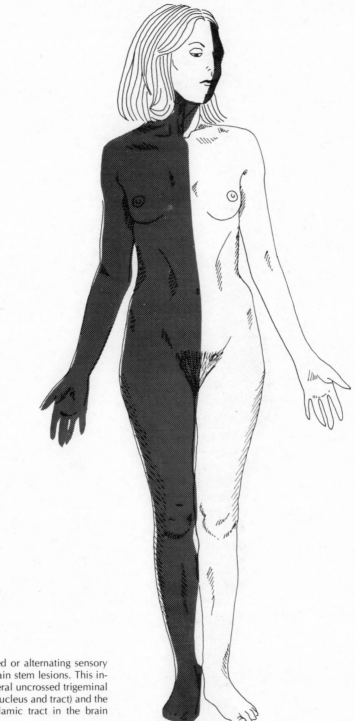

Fig. 4-7B. Crossed or alternating sensory loss seen with brain stem lesions. This involves the ipsilateral uncrossed trigeminal sensory system (nucleus and tract) and the crossed spinothalamic tract in the brain stem.

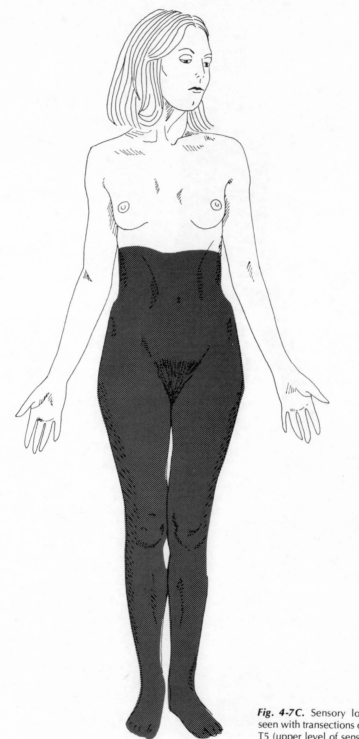

Fig. 4-7C. Sensory loss (all modalities) seen with transections of the spinal cord at T5 (upper level of sensory loss is at T7).

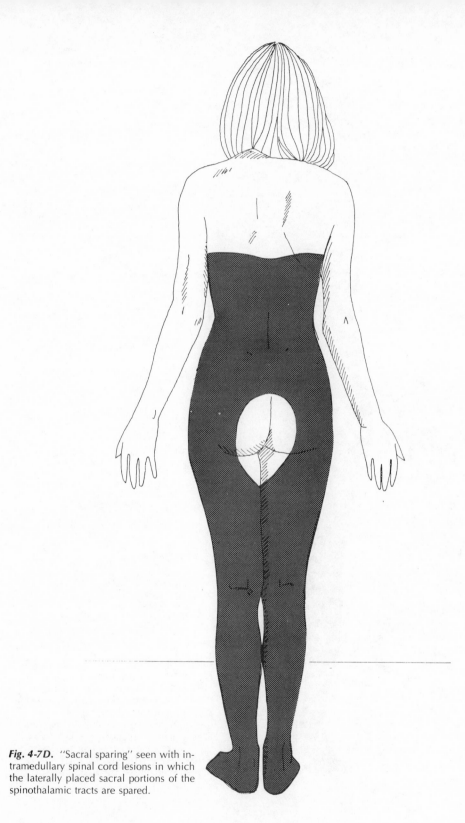

Fig. 4-7D. "Sacral sparing" seen with intramedullary spinal cord lesions in which the laterally placed sacral portions of the spinothalamic tracts are spared.

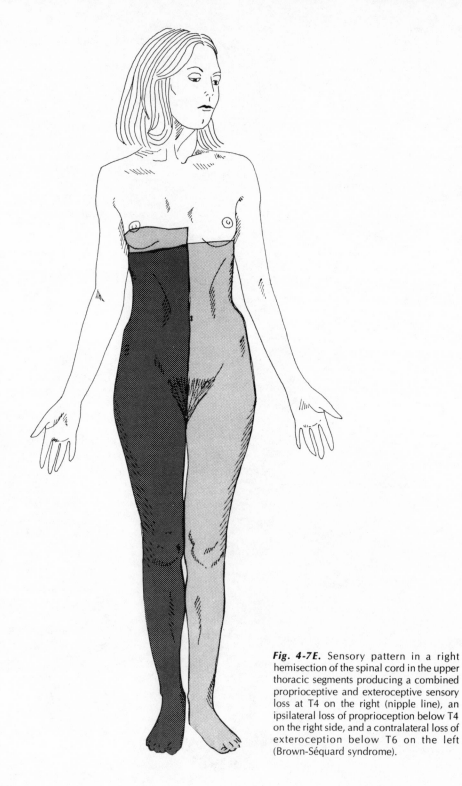

Fig. 4-7E. Sensory pattern in a right hemisection of the spinal cord in the upper thoracic segments producing a combined proprioceptive and exteroceptive sensory loss at T4 on the right (nipple line), an ipsilateral loss of proprioception below T4 on the right side, and a contralateral loss of exteroception below T6 on the left (Brown-Séquard syndrome).

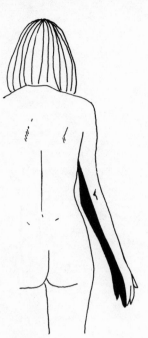

Fig. 4-7F. Radicular sensory loss seen in C8 sensory root lesions

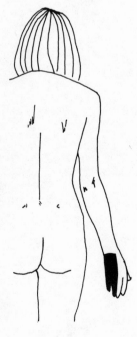

Fig. 4-7G. Peripheral nerve sensory loss seen in ulnar nerve lesions (contrast with C8 pattern).

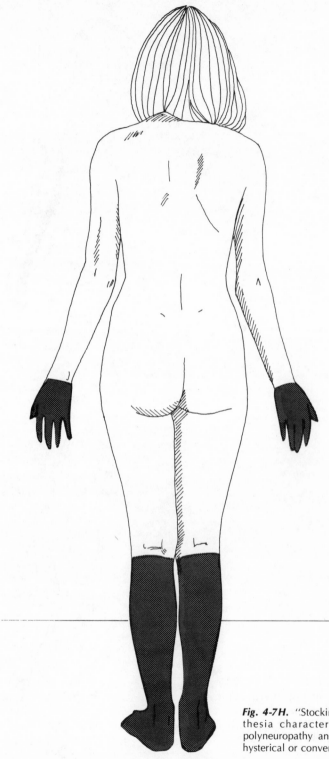

Fig. 4-7H. "Stocking and glove" hypesthesia characteristically seen with polyneuropathy and very rarely seen in hysterical or conversion reactions

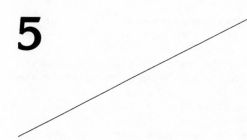

5

THE REFLEXES

STRETCH REFLEXES

The stretch (or deep tendon) reflex is a rapid monosynaptic reflex. It is elicited either by percussing the tendon of a muscle directly or by percussing a part of the body with a reflex hammer in a manner that causes joint movement that will stretch the muscle. A well-balanced hammer with a soft rubber head should be used, one that delivers a firm but soft blow on an area large enough to cause stretching of a muscle tendon. The examiner should deliver a quick, bouncing blow like the strike of a drumstick or the hammer of a piano, not like a hammer driving a nail. This is best accomplished by holding the hammer between the thumb and forefinger distal to the point of balance. It makes little difference whether the reflex hammer is shaped like a wheel, a hammer, or a triangle. The long-handled "Queen Square" hammer delivers an equal blow every time as gravity alone causes it to have adequate momentum to elicit a reflex. The smaller hammers are more convenient to carry.

Lesions of the lower motor neuron (anterior horn cell, motor root, peripheral nerve), primary sensory neuron (posterior root, dorsal root ganglion, peripheral nerve) and spinal cord segment cause these reflexes to decrease or disappear. Lesions of the upper motor neurons (corticospinal, pyramidal, spinal cord internuncial pool) impinging on the lower motor neuron supplying the muscle, cause these reflexes to increase. They may not only increase, but the reflexogenic zone spreads to involve other reflexes. Clonus (see p. 76) may appear with hyperactive reflexes; however, in acute lesions, "spinal shock" may cause these reflexes to be absent initially.

The reflexes throughout the body should be of about the same magnitude and equal on the left and right sides. The method for eliciting stretch reflexes in patients in both the sitting and the supine position is described for most reflexes. The patient must have muscles relaxed with the extremity hanging loosely or resting comfortably. Any muscle tension to maintain posture may artificially increase or decrease the reflex. Minimal reflexes can be brought out or exaggerated by asking the patient to forcefully contract a muscle group not involved in the examination. This is called "Jendrassik reinforcement." The patient can be asked to pull interlocked hands apart, clench the jaw, or squeeze the examiner's arm.

The nerves conducting the nerve impulses for a particular reflex, and the location of the reflex center in the central nervous system, are indicated in the text.

Clonus When the reflexes are very hyperactive, clonus may be elicited by the reflex hammer or by a quick, forceful stretch of the patient's muscle. Clonus is clearly a sign of pathology if it can be sustained indefinitely by maintenance of the tension on the muscle.

It may be helpful to grade the reflexes on the patient's report: 0, no response; 1+, a decreased response; 2+, a normal reflex response; 3+, exaggerated or hyperactive; and 4+, clonus. The examiner should indicate if reinforcement was necessary.

Jaw Reflex—Trigeminal Nerve, Motor Division, Mid Pons The patient keeps the jaw relaxed and slightly opened. The examiner percusses downward on the top of his finger, in a direction that forces the jaw to open (Fig. 5-1).

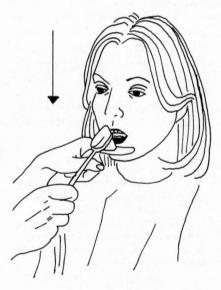

Fig. 5-1. Jaw reflex

Pectoral Reflex—Pectoral Nerves, C6-C8 The patient's arm should be relaxed. The examiner percusses upward against the thumb, which should be tightly pulled up against the pectoralis tendon (Fig. 5-2). Reflex contraction is usually felt, and on occasion can be seen. When these reflexes are both hyperactive, the more active reflex can be elicited by percussing the sternum and observing the bilateral pectoralis contractions to determine which is the greater.

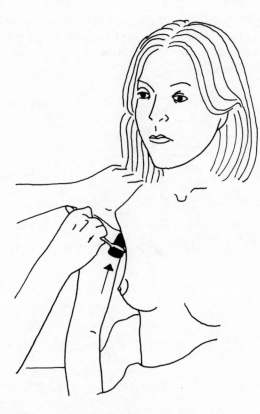

Fig. 5-2. Pectoral reflex

Biceps Reflex—Musculocutaneous Nerve, C5-C6 The thumb or finger is placed against the biceps tendon stretching it slightly (Fig. 5-3) and the thumb is percussed. The tendon's contraction can be felt and usually seen.

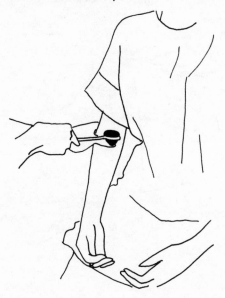

Fig. 5-3. Biceps reflex

Radial Pronator Reflex—Median Nerve, C6-C7 The examiner percusses the radial styloid process on its ventral or palmar surface in a manner that supinates the semipronated wrist (Fig. 5-4). The reflex response causes the wrist to pronate.

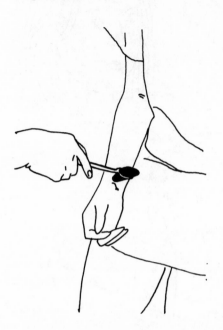

Fig. 5-4. Radial pronator reflex. Examiner hits the radial styloid in a manner that supinates the wrist.

Triceps Reflex—Radial Nerve, C7-C8 The examiner must be sure he hits the tendon of the triceps muscle (Fig. 5-5). It is often valuable to palpate the tendon first, to be sure of its location.

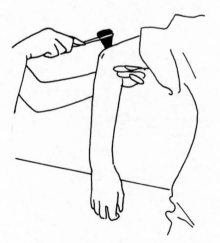

Fig. 5-5. Triceps reflex

Finger Flexion Reflex—Median and Ulnar Nerves, C7-T1 The patient is instructed to hold his fingers in a semiflexed position against the examiner's fingers applied at right angles. The examiner then percusses the dorsum of his fingers (Fig. 5-6). This reflex employs the same reflex arc as the Hoffman reflex but is more efficient. It will show a reflex response with hypoactive reflexes. The Hoffman is present only when this reflex is hyperactive and a spread to the thumb flexors is seen.

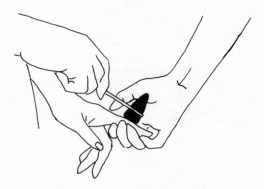

Fig. 5-6. Finger flexion reflex

Deep Abdominal Stretch Reflexes—Intercostal Nerves, T6-T12 This reflex is not to be confused with the superficial abdominal reflex that is part of the cutaneous reflexes (see p. 85). The abdominal muscle is put on a stretch from the costal margins or inguinal ligament by the examiner's hand (Fig. 5-7). The hand is percussed to stretch the muscle; the contraction can be felt. Abdominal relaxation by the patient is essential for eliciting this reflex.

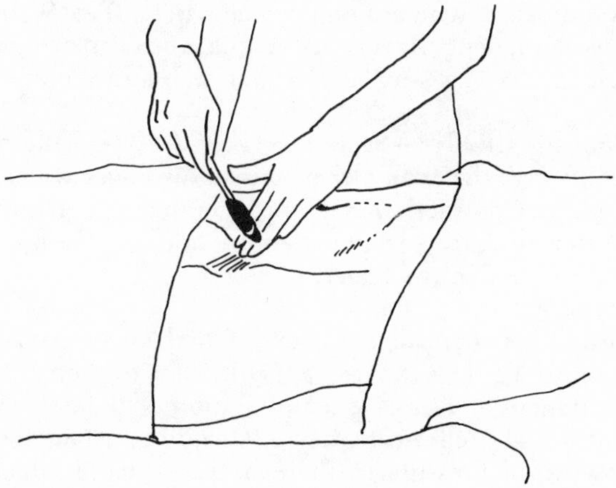

Fig. 5-7. Deep abdominal stretcl
reflex

Puboadductor Reflex—Obturator Nerve, L2-L4 The examiner strikes his hand which is placed on the medial aspect of the knee. The thigh is seen to jerk inwards as the puboadductors contract reflexly. When hyperactive, the puboadductor reflex on the opposite side will also be seen (Fig. 5-8A). With bilaterally hyperactive reflexes, the more hyperactive can be identified by tapping a hand placed on the pubic bone, causing both puboadductor reflexes to react (Fig. 5-8B).

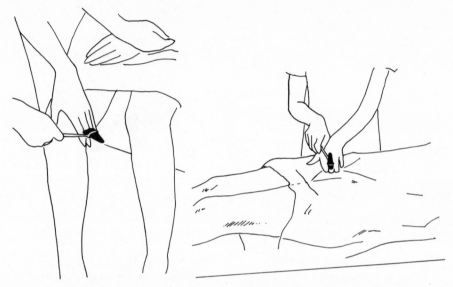

Fig. 5-8. (A) Pubo-adductor reflex; (B) Bilateral pubo-adductor reflex

Patellar (Quadriceps) Reflex—Femoral Nerve, L2-L4 In eliciting this reflex, the examiner should make certain that he has located the tendon and is percussing it squarely with his hammer (Fig. 5-9). On the supine patient, clonus can be sought by a quick downward pull on the patella (Fig. 5-10), stretching the quadriceps muscle suddenly. If very active, the reflex can be muted by percussing above the patella, causing a less efficient stretch and a more easily observed response.

Hamstring Reflex—Sciatic Nerve, L2-L4 On the prone patient with the knee semiflexed, the examiner percusses his finger which is placed on the hamstring tendons. Contraction may be seen, or just felt, in the tendon (Fig. 5-11). This can be elicited in the sitting patient by hooking the hamstring tendon with a finger and percussing the finger.

Ankle (Gastrocnemius) Reflex—Tibial Nerve S1-S2 Two methods are shown in Figure 5-12. This can be a difficult reflex to elicit and requires both relaxation of the patient and passive manipulation of the ankle joint to provide the proper tension. The reflex can often be elicited by asking the patient to give a very slight downward pressure to the examiner's hand which is placed on the plantar surface of the foot. Clonus can be sought by sudden, forcible dorsiflexion of the

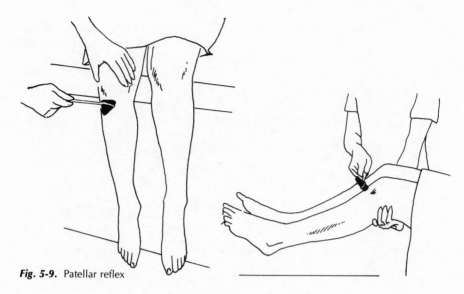

Fig. 5-9. Patellar reflex

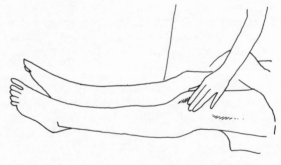

Fig. 5-10. Eliciting patellar clonus

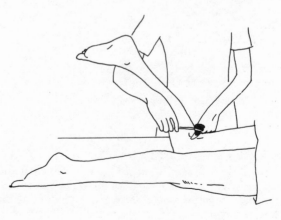

Fig. 5-11. Hamstring reflex

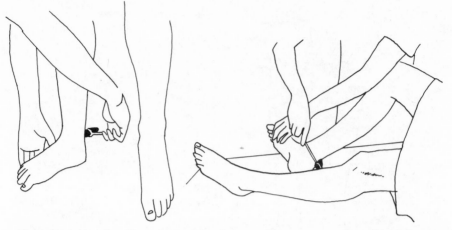

Fig. 5-12. Ankle reflex. The patient puts barely perceptible pressure on the examiner's hand.

foot with the knee partially bent. The ankle jerk can be best obtained on the supine patient by insuring that the knee is slightly flexed. The examiner must exhaust all methods of eliciting this reflex before he considers it absent. Repeated percussion of the belly of the gastrocnemius muscle before eliciting the ankle reflex may facilitate its appearance.

Gluteal Reflex—Gluteal Nerve, L4-S2 The examiner applies a downward pull on the buttock and percusses his fingers (Fig. 5-13). The reflex can usually be felt and sometimes seen.

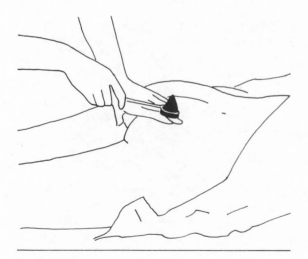

Fig. 5-13. Gluteal reflex

SUPERFICIAL CUTANEOUS REFLEXES

These reflexes are best elicited by a light scratch with a sharp point, applied with increasing force until a response is obtained.

Superficial cutaneous reflexes are polysynaptic and depend upon an intact corticospinal pathway for their normal expression. An abnormal response usually indicates a functional or anatomical lesion of the corticospinal, pyramidal, or upper motor neuron system. The corneal reflex belongs to this group but will be considered with the cranial nerves.

Plantar Reflex The stimulus to elicit this reflex should be sharp, but slowly and gently applied (Fig. 5-14) to the most lateral aspect of the sole of the foot from the heel to the base of the little toe (Fig. 5-15). If no response occurs, the stimulus should be reapplied with slightly more force. The normal response is flexion of the great toe, and sometimes the other toes, or no response at all. The abnormal response (Babinski sign) is extension of the great toe with or without fanning of the toes. (This response is normal in children under 1 to 2 years of age.) Contraction of the extensor hallicus longus tendon must be seen on the dorsal surface of the toe in an extensor or abnormal response.

A withdrawal response can simulate the abnormal extensor plantar reflex in a patient who is sensitive to the stimulus. In this instance, the confirmatory toe signs (see p. 85) are helpful. Also, a sharp stroke or pinch to the dorsum of the foot near the base of the toes can differentiate a withdrawal from an extensor response. With this stimulus a withdrawal would produce plantar flexion of the toes and foot. With an abnormal reflex, plantar extension will occur despite a withdrawal response. The commonest mistakes in eliciting this reflex are failure to use a sharp stimulus, stroking too fast, and stroking too medially on the foot.

The Chaddock, Oppenheim, and Gordon reflexes are referred to as confirmatory toe signs to be used when the plantar response is equivocal, yet expected to be positive. The toe responses in these reflexes are interpreted in the same manner as in the plantar reflex.

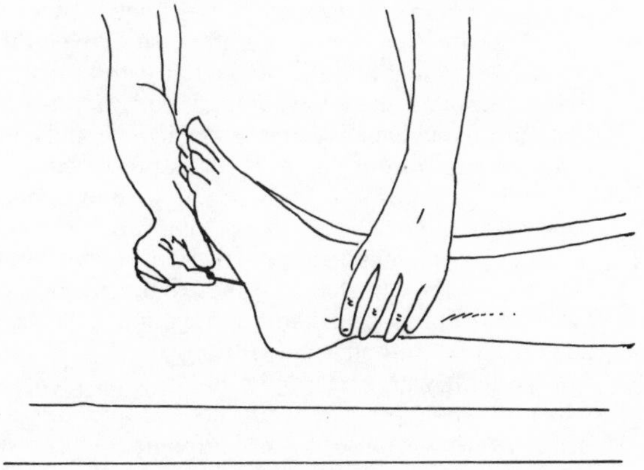

Fig. 5-14. Plantar reflex

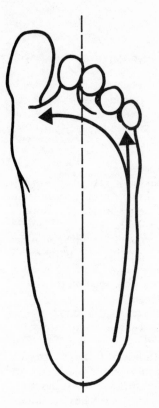

Fig. 5-15. Route that a sharp stimulus should follow, slowly, on the plantar aspect of the foot to elicit the plantar reflex.

Normal plantar flexion is a multiple-stage response often visible only in hyperactive normal individuals, but present on electromyography. It consists of three phases involving flexion of the plantar muscles, dorsiflexion of the foot, and flexion of the knee and thigh. In pathological states with a positive or extensor toe sign, this response is exaggerated. It is then called the "triple flexion response." In the plantar extensor response, early and marked contraction of the tensor fascia lata can be seen on the anterolateral surface of the thigh and can serve as an indication of the pathological reflex. The only difference between the triple flexion response in the normal individual and the individual with an extensor plantar response is that the dorsiflexor of the great toe contracts early and overpowers the plantar flexors of the foot. With involvement of the corticospinal system anywhere in its course, an extensor response of the great toe is produced.

The Babinski response may not be seen in upper motor neuron lesions if there is paralysis of the extensor hallucis longus due to peroneal nerve damage. In chronic paraplegics or hemiplegics, the peroneal nerve can be compressed in bed or against the frame of the wheelchair. Although the extensor plantar response (Babinski) is the hallmark of corticospinal tract dysfunction, it can be seen in sleep, after anesthesia, in fatigue states, and after convulsions.

In patients with frontal lobe lesions, the plantar stimulus may produce a grasp reflex inhibiting an extensor response in the toe. The Chaddock stimulus does not evoke a grasp response. As a consequence, a flexor plantar response, but a positive or extensor Chaddock response, may point to a frontal lobe lesion.

Chaddock Reflex The stimulus is applied to the lateral aspect of the foot, starting around the ankle and carried up to the lateral aspect of the little toe.

Oppenheim Reflex A strong rub in one stroke, proximal to distal, on the skin overlying the tibia.

Gordon Reflex A firm squeeze of the lower leg and gastrocnemius in an anterior-posterior direction.

Superficial Abdominal Reflex This reflex requires a quick, light, long, brisk stroke with a pin over the skin of the four quadrants of the abdominal wall (Fig. 5-16). The normal response is a contraction of the abdominal wall under the stimulus, causing the umbilicus to move to the side stroked. The abnormal manifestation is usually no response, or it can be a strong, delayed response involving more of the lateral abdominal wall than is usually noted. Total absence of the abdominal reflex bilaterally may be of no significance. It is usually absent in obese patients and in those who are pregnant. The abdominal reflex is most significant when present on one side but not on the other. This is a sign of corticospinal tract involvement.

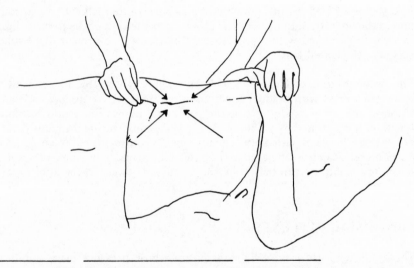

Fig. 5-16. Superficial abdominal reflex

Superficial Gluteal Reflex Total absence of the gluteal reflex may be of no significance. It is significant of corticospinal tract damage when present on one side but not on the other. A quick stroke over the skin of the buttock produces visible contraction (Fig. 5-17).

Cremasteric Reflex The cremasteric reflex can be elicited in the male by a firm pin stroke up the upper inner thigh, causing ipsilateral withdrawal of the scrotum due to cremasteric muscle contraction. Unilateral absence indicates corticospinal tract involvement.

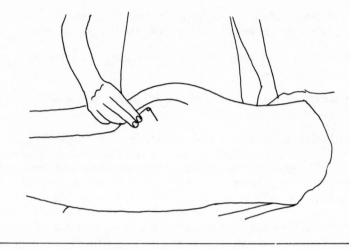

Fig. 5-17. Superficial gluteal reflex

Anal Reflex—S3-S5 Contraction of the anal ring is either felt with the introduction of the fingertip into the anus or observed as the skin of the perineal area is scratched or pricked with a pin. Absence indicates involvement of peripheral nerves of the spinal cord.

The Bulbocavernosus Reflex—S3-S4 This reflex is valuable in assessing the reflexes involved with bladder function in paraplegics. Its absence indicates a lesion in the conus medullaris or the peripheral nerves important to bladder function. It is initiated by pinching the foreskin, compressing the glans penis, or pricking the foreskin with a pin. The response, a contraction of the bulbocavernosus muscle, can be seen or felt at the base of the penis. In women, a response to pinching the clitoris can be felt by the examiner's finger in the anal canal.

ABNORMAL REFLEXES

These reflexes form a miscellaneous group whose presence usually indicates diffuse cerebral cortical dysfunction or bilateral frontal lobe involvement.

Grasp Reflex in the Hand This reflex consists of an involuntary grasp of the examiner's hand as a result of stroking the palm of the patient's hand. The examiner's stroke begins on the volar surface of the wrist (Fig. 5-18A) and extends into the palm (Fig. 5-18B) past the palmar surfaces of the fingertips. The patient should be instructed not to grasp voluntarily. It is usually found with contralateral frontal lobe dysfunction.

> Several degrees of grasp reflex in the fingers may be noted from a simple hooking of the fingers to a forceful grasp strong enough to allow the examiner to pull the patient out of bed.

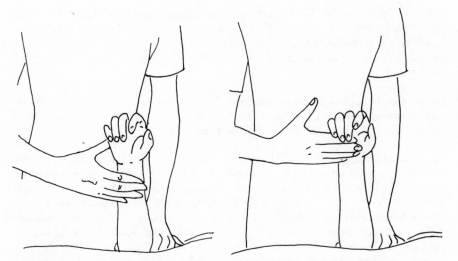

Fig. 5-18. Method for eliciting grasp reflex in hand. *(A)* Beginning, and *(B)* in progress

Grasp Reflex of the Foot This is elicited by pressure on the ball of the foot with a blunt stimulus brought up through the center of the sole (Fig. 5-19). Forcible flexion of all the toes in a grasping movement is seen with contralateral frontal lobe lesion.

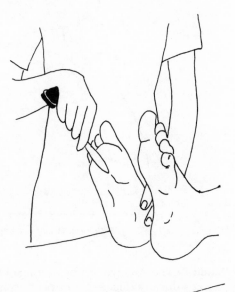

Fig. 5-19. Method for eliciting grasp reflex in the foot

Groping or Forced Groping of the Hand This rare reflex is usually seen in patients with a contralateral frontal lobe lesion, and rarely in those with a deep ipsilateral frontal lobe lesion. The sight of the examiner's hand near the patient's hand, or a slight stroke between the patient's thumb and first finger, can cause forced movements of the patient's hand in a sequence of movements aimed at grabbing the stimulus. Such forced movements of the arm and hand can sometimes be seen when an object (*e.g.*, a percussion hammer) is dangled in front of the patient.

Groping or Forced Groping in the Foot   This is elicited by a light stroke of the medial margin of the great toe. The patient's foot shows forced movement toward the stimulus with flexion of the toes.

Myerson (Glabellar) Reflex   This reflex consists of an involuntary, usually forceful, repeated orbicularis oculi contraction as the result of a repeated tap on the glabella (Fig. 5-20). The patient is instructed to keep his eyes open. When marked, this reflex can appear as the examiner percusses the midforehead and slowly approaches the glabella. This abnormal reflex is seen in parkinsonism, diffuse cortical disease, and in bilateral frontal lobe lesions. An ipsilateral increase in this reflex can be seen with intrapontine lesions affecting the corticobulbar fibers. An ipsilateral decrease can be seen in patients with nuclear lesions of nerve VII. This response can be seen transiently in tense or anxious patients. Only a persistent response can be considered abnormal.

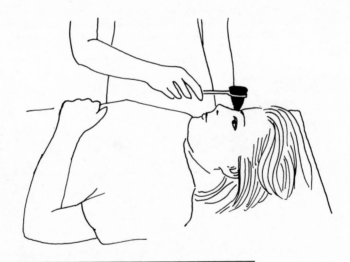

Fig. 5-20. Method for eliciting glabellar reflex (Myerson)

Snout Reflex   An involuntary pursing of the lips is seen following percussion of the lips directly (Fig. 5-21) or percussion transmitted through a tongue blade lying across the lips. This reflex is seen in patients with diffuse, usually frontal, cortical disease.

Suck Reflex   An involuntary sucking movement of the lips, stimulated by an object such as the end of a tongue blade drawn across the lips, can be seen in

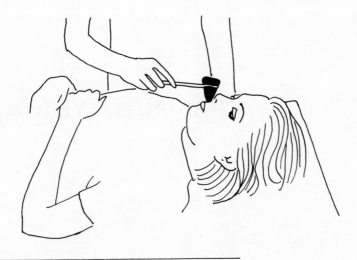

Fig. 5-21. A method for eliciting snout reflex

patients with severe, diffuse cortical disease. Unilateral occurrence of this reflex can point to contralateral frontal lobe involvement.

Palmomental Reflex Contraction of the mentalis muscle in the midline of the lower lip can be seen on forceful stroking of the palm with a sharp stimulus. This reflex is seen transiently in anxious or normal persons, but is persistent in those with diffuse cortical or frontal lobe disease. It can be seen contralateral to unilateral frontal lobe disease.

Sensory examination requires interpretation by the patient, and the motor examination requires cooperation of the patient. Information gained from the reflex examination has the advantage of objectivity since the patient can do little to alter the response. Since the stretch reflexes provide an excellent survey of sensory and motor nerve function, the function of segmental levels of the nervous system, and the superficial cutaneous reflexes assay corticospinal function, the results of these examinations should be correlated with the results of motor and sensory dysfunction patterns seen in the patient. This section on reflex examination was deliberately placed after both the sensory and motor examinations to remind the reader that reflexes test both systems. Altered reflexes may indicate neural dysfunction prior to any sensory or motor disabilities.

6

CRANIAL NERVE SYSTEMS

The examinations discussed in this chapter test not only the intactness of the cranial nerves and their nuclei, but also the intactness of the supranuclear central nervous system pathways that influence the cranial nerves. Therefore, care should always be taken to determine, if possible, whether any abnormalities presented by the patient are due to damage in the cranial nerve, nucleus, or supranuclear pathway.

CRANIAL NERVE I

Smell

The patient's nose should first be examined for obstruction, mucus, or inflammation that would affect the results. The examiner should test only one nostril at a time. He should block one nostril before presenting an odor to the other nostril, and should not release the nostril until after the patient has indicated he has smelled the odor and has identified it, if possible. It is important to use nonirritant odors (*e.g.,* coffee, soap, chewing gum, tobacco, clove). Mucosal irritants (*e.g.,* alcohol, ammonia, and other volatile substances) stimulate sensation by way of cranial nerve V.

> Unilateral loss of smell can be seen in patients with olfactory groove meningiomas, deep frontal lobe tumors, and fractures of the anterior fossa of the skull.

CRANIAL NERVE II

Confrontation

Confrontation testing is the most convenient way of surveying for the intactness of the visual fields. For this examination, one of the patient's eyes should be covered with a card, occluder, eyepatch, or the patient's or examiner's hand, and the patient should not be able to see through cracks at the edges of any occluder used. The patient is then asked to fix his other eye steadily on the examiner's nose; during the examination, the examiner should watch the patient's eye constantly to make sure that fixation is not lost.

The examiner should use a test object of a color easily contrasted from the background and at least one centimeter in diameter or width. The examiner's index finger can be used, or such objects as the head of a large hat pin or cap of a pen. A white and red object of the same size allows the examiner to quantitate the degree of visual field loss as red perception is affected by very minimal visual field defects.

The object selected by the examiner is then slowly moved from the far periphery of the patient's visual field inwards in four quadrants (above, below, right, left). The patient is asked to state when he first becomes aware of the object's presence. It is helpful to wiggle the object slightly as it is moved into the visual field. Since the patient's temporal field is extensive, the examiner should start with the object on the lateral side of the patient's head, as far back as the ear (Fig. 6-1).

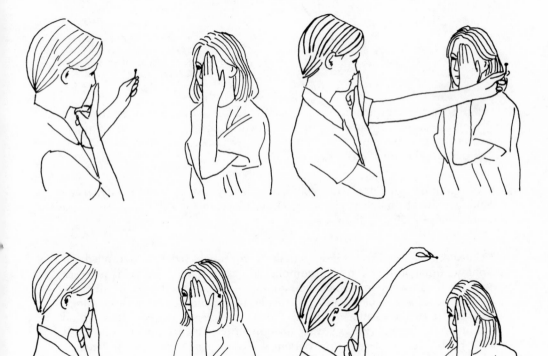

Fig. 6-1. Confrontation testing. Examiner is bringing in a stimulus from beyond the patient's field of vision to many positions around the patient's field.

If there is doubt about the fullness of the visual field on confrontation testing, the patient should be asked to count fingers bilaterally presented in each of the four quadrants (Fig. 6-2). Challenge him with the identification of varying numbers of fingers on one and both hands. If a relative defect (opposed to an absolute defect) is present, the patient may be able to see the object when the individual fields are challenged, but he may not be able to count correctly how many are present when both fields are challenged simultaneously (see p. 93).

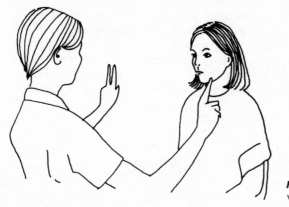

Fig. 6-2. Testing of simultaneous visual fields

An apparent contraction of the visual fields from above may be due to a prominent brow. Tilt the head of the patient slightly backward to eliminate brows as a possible source of erroneous interpretation. Similarly, a large nose can obscure the lower nasal field.

Confrontation with Poor Acuity With remarkably reduced visual acuity, visual fields can still be established by using a large object that is well illuminated, or a bright image such as a flashlight.

Confrontation by Threat If a patient is confused, sedated, obtunded, or aphasic, often all that can be accomplished in checking visual fields is to see whether the patient blinks when the examiner's fist is thrust into each half of the visual field. It is possible to pick up gross homonymous defects in this manner. The thrust of the examiner's hand should not create a breeze that would stimulate the corneal reflex. In very uncooperative patients, intact visual fields may be inferred by seeing if the patient will glance at a bright or threatening object presented suddenly in a peripheral field.

Formal visual field testing with tangent screen and perimetry is indicated in patient's with a possible supratentorial lesion on clinical examination; unexplained loss of vision; a demonstrable field defect on confrontation testing, unless such a defect is readily explained by, for example, a detached retina; papilledema (not so much to chart the size of the blind spot as to look for a possible localizing defect); an enlarged sella turcica seen on radiograph; and any obscure neurological diagnostic problem.

Simultaneous Visual Fields

Presenting stimuli in both visual fields with the patient's eyes open can often disclose defects not easily elicited by individual field testing. This is especially true with deep parietal lobe lesions affecting the visual pathways (see the discussion of simultaneous sensory testing on p. 57). A convenient method is to ask the patient to total the number of fingers flashed quickly in both visual fields by the examiner (see Fig. 6-2). The examiner should flash the fingers for only a fraction of a second and then close his fist. He must be certain the patient is fixing his eyes straight ahead at the examiner's nose.

Ishihara pseudoisochromatic cards for color blindness can also reveal *← due to red perception prob* homonymous field losses if the patient fails to describe either the left- or right-hand numbers consistently in the two number tests.

The visual fields are very sensitive to red. An early homonymous field loss may be detected by presenting two identical red objects (or the palms of both hands) to the left and right of the patient's center of vision (the examiner's nose) and asking if they are identical in color. The patient should look only at the examiner's nose and not at the objects themselves. If one object appears darker than the other it suggests a homonymous field loss. (The color of the walls behind the examiner must be uniform).

Mapping Scotoma

Scotoma (see p. 94) can be detected by asking the patient whether there are any holes or defects in his vision when he looks at the examiner or at a printed text with one eye covered. A central scotoma creates an obvious hole, spot, or visual defect in the center of vision. Other scotoma may not be noted by the patient, since central acuity is not involved and the brain tends to fill in holes in the peripheral fields of one eye. For example, with one eye closed, you are not aware of your own blind spot unless an object is deliberately moved into it and it disappears. Therefore, in the same manner, the patient is asked to look at the examiner's nose and to report whether he can see the examiner's hair, ears, chin, shoulders, or other part of his body. While the patient is still looking at the nose, a red object can be moved about the visual field and the patient is asked if it disappears or decreases in color intensity.

Mapping the Blind Spot

The blind spot can be mapped by the examiner if he covers one eye of the patient (or asks the patient to cover one eye) and closes his own eye opposite that of the patient's closed eye. He then asks the patient to stare at the examiner's open eye. In this way, the examiner can be certain that the patient's gaze does not deviate, and that it lines up the examiner's blind spot opposite the patient's for comparison. The examiner should use a small ball on a pin, 5 mm or less, and place it in his own blind spot at approximately 20° temporally from fixation. He then moves it slowly toward and away from the patient, keeping it in his own blind spot, until it enters the patient's blind spot and is seen by the patient to disappear. The blind spot is caused by the light-insensitive nerve head (optic disc) that sits in the nasal side of the macula in the light-sensitive retina.

The size of the blind spot can be estimated against the size of the examiner's by moving the pin in many different directions from the center of the blind spot to determine when it reappears. Enlargement of the blind spot is seen in patients with engorgement of the nerve head (papilledema), but it does not tend to occur with inflammation of the nerve head (papillitis). Both can look similar on ophthalmoscopy. Scotomata can also be mapped by this technique.

Visual Field Pathology (Anatomical Correlation)

Figure 6-3 is a diagrammatic representation of the base of the brain showing the two ocular globes, the optic nerves, optic chiasm, optic tracts surrounding the mid-brain of the brain stem, geniculate bodies, geniculocalcarine radiations (visual radiations), and occipital visual cortex (calcarine cortex).

The term "hemianopsia" refers to half field defects. Homonymous hemianopsia is the involvement of the same half field in both eyes. Homonymous hemianopsia can be "congruous" (similar) or incongruous. Quadrantanopsia is quarter field involvement. These defects are usually seen in patients with lesions behind the optic chiasm. When the patient has a homonymous field defect, the examiner knows the lesion is behind the chiasm, but the exact location may be impossible to differentiate.

The term "scotoma" refers to areas of visual defect within the field of vision usually caused by retinal or optic nerve lesions. They can be positive if the patient sees a dark spot, or negative if there is no visual image similar to the field defect of the normal blind spot. Constriction of the periphery of the fields can be seen with optic nerve lesions and long-standing chronic papilledema. The right visual field of both eyes (solid lines) stimulates the left retinae of both eyes; conversely, the left visual field stimulates the right retinae (dotted lines in Fig. 6-3). The crossing of nasal retinal fibers and noncrossing of temporal retinal fibers ensures that the right visual fields are represented on the left visual cortex (solid lines).

This is a gross simplification of the visual apparatus. Further study in this area is clinically rewarding.

Figure 6-4 shows five diagrammatic representations of visual field abnormalities associated with visual system lesions in several crucial areas shown in Figure 6-3.

1. Optic nerve lesions cause a unilateral visual loss.
2. Chiasmatic lesions may classically cause a bitemporal hemianopsia (many varieties of field loss are possible).
3. Lesions anywhere from the chiasm to the occipital cortex can produce a homonymous hemianopsia. Optic tract lesions produce a contralateral homonymous hemianopsia without macular sparing and typical incongruous fields.
4. Temporal lobe lesions may involve the inferior retinal radiations that move far anteriorly into the temporal lobe. This can cause a superior, contralateral quadrantanopsia.
5. Occipital lobe lesions can produce a contralateral homonymous hemianopsia with macular sparing (preservation of central lesion).

Visual Acuity

In good illumination, the patient's ability to read small type at a distance of 14 inches from each eye should be estimated. The Jaeger test card, the AMA reading card, or similar cards with standardized type will allow for accurate assessment

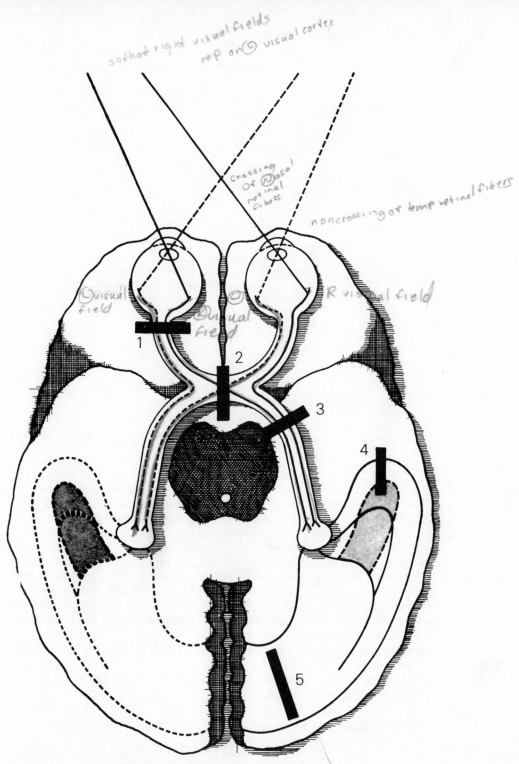

so that right visual fields rep on ① visual cortex

crossing of Ⓝasal retinal fibers

noncrossing or temp retinal fibers

Ⓛ visual field

Ⓝ Ⓛ visual field

R visual field

1

2

3

4

5

Fig. 6-3. Diagram of visual pathways (see text)

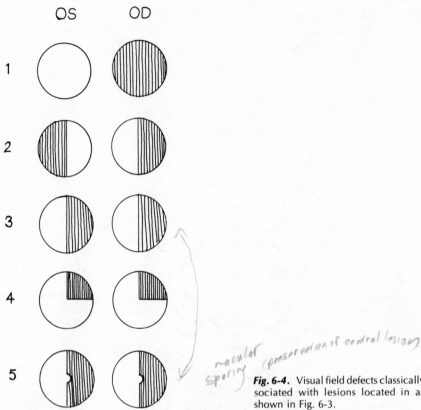

OS   OD

1

2

3

4

5

macular sparing (preservation of central lesion)

Fig. 6-4. Visual field defects classically associated with lesions located in areas shown in Fig. 6-3.

of change on repeated examination, or correlation between examiners. However, small print, as in a book or magazine, can be substituted if charts are not available. The examiner should record both the approximate size of the type used and the smallest type that can be read by the patient with infrequent errors.

Loss of visual acuity due to optic nerve involvement is of importance in the neurological examination. Therefore, loss of acuity on any other basis, such as, refractive error, should be minimized. The examination should be performed with the patient's glasses. If the visual acuity is reduced, and glasses are not available, a pinhole may be used to neutralize the loss of acuity due to uncorrected refractive error or irregularities in the ocular media. Use of the pinhole requires good illumination of the target.

The manner in which the letters are read by the patient may help to indicate the presence of a visual field defect. For example, if a patient reads only the left-hand letters with the right eye, and the right-hand letters with the left eye, a bitemporal hemianopsia could be suspected.

Ophthalmoscopic Examination

The ocular fundus must be carefully examined, if at all possible, in every patient. The examiner should develop skill in examining fundi without dilating the pupil. Dilating the pupil with a mydriatic should be reserved for extensive retinal examination or when the fundus cannot be seen because of opacities. Mydriatics should never be used in patients with impending cerebral dysfunction in which a dilating pupil would be an important sign. In evaluating the optic disc and the macula, each of the four retinal quadrants should be surveyed systematically. The examiner should learn to recognize:

1. Papilledema, especially early.
2. Optic atrophy.
3. Hemorrhages and exudates.
4. Retinal arteriolar changes of hypertension.
5. Vascular changes of diabetes.
6. Degenerative retinal changes such as chorioretinitis (healed and active) and retinitis pigmentosa.

For this examination, the examiner should have the patient fix the eyes on a well-defined, easily seen, small object across a darkened room. The patient's right eye should be examined with the examiner's right; the patient's left eye with the examiner's left eye. The examiner's head should not block the object the patient is looking at for fixation (Fig. 6-5).

Wandering fixation, as seen in young children, may make the ophthalmoscopic examination difficult. If the patient has reduced vision, fixation can be obtained by asking him to look in the direction of his finger held out in front, his gaze directed by proprioceptive information.

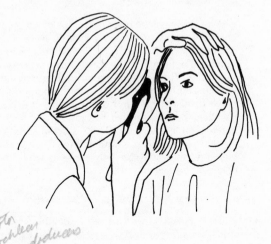

Fig. 6-5. Use of the ophthalmoscope

CRANIAL NERVES III, IV, VI (OCULOMOTOR SYSTEM)

Pupillary Light Reflex

The pupils should react briskly and equally to light, both directly (eye stimulated) and consensually (opposite). When testing the direct light reflex, the examiner should be certain the light is not diffusing into the opposite eye. With dark irises, the consensual reflex can be seen by transilluminating the pupil with a soft light (ophthalmoscope light) from the side, in a position that does not produce a pupillary reflex.

Disorders Causing Alterations of the Pupillary Reflex to Light

Argyll Robertson pupil: Loss of response to light, direct and consensually with a normal response to convergence and accommodation (see below). This is often associated with miosis and pupillary irregularity. It is most frequently seen in patients with neurosyphilis.

Tonic pupil (Adie's pupil): Slow or abolished response to light and darkness, as well as convergence. Both contraction and dilation are involved in this pupillary anomaly.

Internal ophthalmoplegia: A paralytic mydriasis associated with lesions of cranial nerve III, especially when it is compressed behind the cavernous venous sinus by herniation of the tip of the temporal lobe through the incisura of the cerebellar tentorium in cerebral edema.

Amaurotic pupillary paresis: With destruction of the optic nerve or retina, and severe unilateral blindness, the pupils will not respond directly or consensually to light in the blind eye. Both pupils will respond to light in the intact eye.

Hemianopic pupillary paralysis: With lesions of the optic tract producing a hemianopsia, response of both pupils is absent or diminished when finely focused light enters the pupils from the hemianopic fields. (Many feel that this response is more fiction than fact. Find out for yourself.)

Swinging Flashlight Test In minimal or old optic nerve lesions where visual acuity may be intact, a paradoxical apparent dilation of the pupil, on stimulation with the flashlight, can be seen if the flashlight is swung from one eye to the other in an alternating fashion. The rate of swing may have to be varied to elicit the paradoxical dilatation.

> With lesions of the optic nerve, the direct pupillary response is affected in this test, but the consensual remains intact. With minimal optic nerve damage, the afferent stimulus for pupillary constriction will not be transmitted as efficiently by way of the ipsilateral optic nerve (direct route) as through the contralateral optic nerve (consensual route). The flashlight provides the same stimulus intensity to both eyes, and by swinging it provides the same short stimulus duration. Therefore, with minimal optic nerve damage, the pupil of the involved eye seems to enlarge in the face of the flashlight stimulation that has just swung back from stimulating the normal optic nerve of the consensual eye. Its dilation in the face of a light stimulus is a readjustment to a less efficient stimulus. If the flashlight lingers, the pupil will again constrict; therefore, this sign can only be seen while the light is swinging back and forth between the eyes.

Pupillary Reaction to Near Vision: Accommodation, Convergence

The patient is asked to look at a specific object in the distance. The examiner then places his finger in the patient's line of sight near the patient's face and asks him to look at his finger. This causes accommodation, convergence, and a pupillary constriction that can be clearly seen. Paralysis of convergence can be seen with dorsal midbrain lesions affecting the anterior medial longitudinal fasciculus.

Examination for Ptosis

On forward gaze, the patient's upper eyelid margins should cut across the iris at the same point bilaterally (Fig. 6-6). Ptosis is suspected when one upper lid cuts across the iris at a lower level than the other eye, or when the patient chronically

Fig. 6-6. The examiner must note the position of the upper and lower lids relative to the iris and compare both sides.

tilts the head backward to see, or has chronically raised eyebrows. The examiner should attempt to determine the cause of ptosis. Ptosis can be considered either "partial" or "complete."

Causes for Ptosis

Local pathology (false ptosis)
    Enophthalmos (phthisis bulbi)
    Lid swelling (chalazion)
Sympathetic dysfunction (Horner's syndrome)
    In addition to ptosis, any or all of the following may be observed:
        Disappearance or lessening of the ptosis on upward gaze
            (valuable confirmatory signs for sympathetic ptosis)
        No loss of the upper eyelid fold (as in oculomotor ptosis)
        A reduction of less than 3 mm in the size of the palpebral aperture
            (compared to the other side)
        Small reacting pupil
        Enophthalmos
        Anhydrosis, ipsilateral of the face
Oculomotor paresis
    In addition to ptosis on forward gaze, the following may or may not be seen:
        Persistent ptosis on upward gaze
        Dilated, poorly-reacting or nonreacting pupil
        Partial external ophthalmoplegia
Apparent Ptosis (erroneously labelled pseudoptosis)
    An optical illusion of ptosis occurs when the contralateral palpebral fissure is wider due to facial paresis on that side. In this instance, the lower lid is also seen to be higher on what is really the normal side.
Myopathic or Myasthenic Ptosis
    In myopathy of the extraocular muscles, one would expect to see other evidence of myopathy or myasthenia. The muscle involvement may not follow any neurogenic pattern.

Ocular Motility on Following Examiner's Finger (Pursuit Movements)

The examiner moves his finger in a manner that will test all directions of gaze (right, left, up, down, obliquely) and test convergence (Fig. 6-7). He observes the patient's eyes for evidence of restricted motility or dysconjugate movement. The examiner should ask the patient if he sees two fingers instead of one (diplopia). Ocular motility can also be tested in each eye separately by covering the other eye. The examiner may be able to observe restricted eye movements in directions of gaze that will implicate paresis of certain extraocular muscles. The presence of

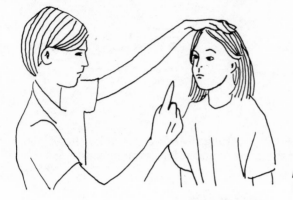

Fig. 6-7. Ocular motility on following the finger

diplopia suggests paresis of one of the paired extraocular muscles active in the direction of the gaze in which diplopia occurs. The examiner must take care that he does not put his fingers too close to the patient's face, causing convergence and confusing eye movements by producing a terminal nystagmoid movement on lateral gaze.

Ocular Motility on Voluntary Gaze (Refixation, Saccadic Movements)

The examiner asks the patient to gaze in all directions voluntarily. If dysconjugate gaze is seen, or diplopia noted by the patient, muscle paresis due to a cranial nerve or muscle disease is implied. The examiner should determine the direction in which diplopia becomes most marked and in which direction it disappears or is minimal (refer to the red glass test, p. 105). Paresis of conjugate gaze, as opposed to paresis in one eye, implicates supranuclear dysfunction.

> With acute or massive lesions of the internal capsule, the patient may not be able to gaze to the contralateral side, or may demonstrate a fixed deviation of the eyes to the side of the lesion. These phenomena often clear in a few days as ipsilateral supranuclear innervation takes over. Paralysis of vertical gaze suggests a lesion involving the midbrain tectum or dorsal pontomedullary area. Paresis of upward gaze can be seen as an associated finding in old age and parkinsonism. Initial paresis of downward gaze can be an early manifestation of generalized supranuclear cerebral degeneration. Paralysis of lateral pursuit movements and intact voluntary or refixation movements may suggest an occipital lobe lesion on the contralateral side to the pursuit paralysis.

Doll's Eye Phenomenon

In upward gaze paresis, the patient may not be able to look upward voluntarily, but will be able to look upward when asked to follow the examiner's finger upward, or if he is asked to fix on the examiner's finger and if his head is passively flexed, causing upward gaze to occur reflexly (Fig. 6-8). This difference

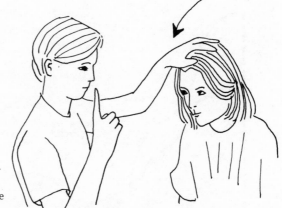

Fig. 6-8. Method of eliciting the "doll's eye" movement

suggests involvement of supranuclear pathways in vertical gaze (see p. 45). The term "Doll's Eye Phenomenon" has often been used incorrectly in referring to the side-to-side gaze movements on head turning (oculocephalic reflex movements).

DISTURBANCES IN GAZE MECHANISMS

Frontal lobe lesions (around Brodmann area 8) may cause a supranuclear gaze paresis to the opposite side. However, the eyes may be able to follow the examiner's fingers. Rarely, lesions of the occipital lobe may cause a paralysis of the following pursuit eye movements to the contralateral side on gaze testing, with voluntary or refixation gaze intact. Bilateral frontal lesions (area 8) of midbrain-posterior third ventricle can affect vertical gaze.

Internuclear ophthalmoplegia is seen with lesions of the medial longitudinal fasciculus between the nuclei of cranial nerves III and VI. On lateral conjugate gaze, the adducting eye does not fully adduct, and the abducting eye may manifest nystagmus. In essence, this is a weakness of lateral conjugate gaze manifested unequally in two lateral rotators. The commonest causes are multiple sclerosis and small areas of softening secondary to vascular insufficiency in the brain stem.

THE EXTRAOCULAR MUSCLES

It is important that the examiner understand the directions of gaze produced by these extraocular muscles. Figure 6-9 shows the characteristic position of the extraocular muscles as they are applied to the eyeball to rotate the globe. It is important to note that the abducted eye (position AB) has its axis parallel to the superior and inferior rectus muscles (SR and IR) which elevate and depress the globe in the abducted position. When the eye is adducted (AD), the axis of the eyeball is parallel to the superior and inferior oblique muscles (SO and IO) which elevate and depress the globe in the adducted position. When the eye is in forward gaze, its axis is between the planes of action of these muscles. Elevation and depression require their combined activities. Figure 6-10 shows the muscles involved in eye movements based on the description above. Knowledge of these patterns will allow the examiner to easily interpret ocular palsies, corneal light reflex, and red glass tests.

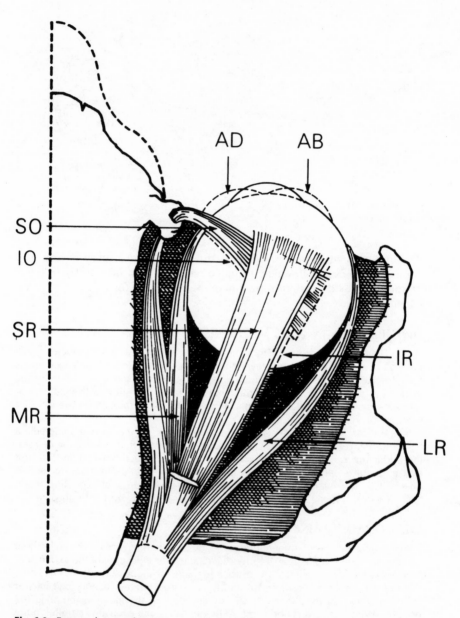

Fig. 6-9. Extraocular muscles. *AB,* eye in abducted position; *AD,* eye in adducted position; *IO,* inferior oblique muscle; *IR,* inferior rectus muscle; *LR,* lateral rectus muscle; *MR,* medial rectus muscle; *SR,* superior rectus muscle; *SO,* superior oblique muscle.

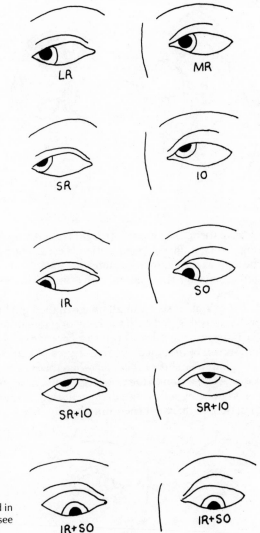

Fig. 6-10. Extraocular muscles involved in various conjugate eye movements (see legend for Fig. 6-9) paired?

Corneal Light Reflex

The patient may have dysconjugate gaze as a result of paresis of the extraocular muscles and yet not complain of diplopia. This can be due to poor visual acuity in one eye, opacities of the cornea or lens in one eye, or long-standing diplopia with subsequent suppression of the image of one eye (amblyopia ex anopsia). The latter is more likely to occur in younger patients than in older ones. Also, the patient may have a dysconjugate gaze that is not gross enough to be appreciated by the examiner who is looking at the patient's ocular movements.

The corneal light reflex examination allows the examiner to detect very small degrees of oculomotor paresis without the need of a subjective report on the part

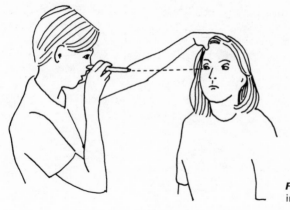

Fig. 6-11. Corneal light reflex testing

of the patient. The examiner sights down a flashlight, as if it were a gun barrel (Fig. 6-11), pointing at the patient's eyes. The patient is asked to fix the eyes on the light as the examiner rotates the patient's head from side to side and up and down, causing the eyes to move in all directions of gaze while fixating on the light.

The examiner sees a small image of the light bulb reflecting from the center of both pupils (Fig. 6-12). If the reflection remains in the center of both pupils with eye movement in all directions of gaze, normal conjugate gaze without muscle paresis can be assumed. A small degree of oculomotor paresis can be detected if the light image shifts off center when the eyes rotate in the direction of gaze that requires the action of the weakened muscle (see red glass test below). Because the eye is not being fully rotated, the reflected image moves off center in the direction of action of the weakened muscle (Fig. 6-13).

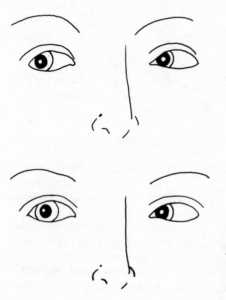

Fig. 6-12. Corneal light seen in a patient with normal ocular motility

Fig. 6-13. Corneal light seen in a patient with right lateral rectus paresis. Reflection in the right cornea is laterally deviated because the eye is lagging behind on abduction.

Concomitant strabismus due to congenital muscle imbalance might mislead the examiner by showing a light reflex off the center in one eye. However, unlike neurogenic paresis, the light reflection remains off center to exactly the same degree in all directions of gaze, including forward gaze. In neurological dysfunction, the image moves more off center as the eye is rotated in the direction of action of the involved muscle. For example, in patients with left lateral rectus palsy, the image of the examiner's light is shifted to the lateral margin of the left pupil when the patient's head is turned to the right.

Red Glass Test

This is a very helpful method to detect paresis of extraocular muscles and to identify the ocular muscles and nerves involved. It is relatively free of error in interpretation. In this test, one eye is covered with a red lens and the patient is asked to look at a bright light source (*e.g.,* a pen light or a candle flame) that is slowly moved in all directions of gaze. This test allows the patient with extraocular paresis to see double more easily. The patient is asked to describe the amount of separation of the two images and their position relative to each other (*i.e.,* separated horizontally, vertically, or diagonally). Frequently, a patient will have diplopia with the red glass that was not otherwise apparent, as the red glass creates dissimilar color images, decreasing the need for binocular fusion.

If, for example, the red glass is placed over the right eye, the examiner is now able to identify the image seen with each eye by the color reported by the patient with diplopia. The red image observed by the patient will always be that seen by the right eye, and the white light will be that seen by the left eye. By moving the light through the various directions of gaze, and asking the patient to follow it with his eyes, the examiner can then determine in which direction separation of the images or diplopia is produced. He should determine whether the separation is horizontal, vertical, or both, and the relative degree of separation as estimated by the patient in inches or centimeters. The examiner can then determine in which direction of gaze the diplopia worsens. If the diplopia is both horizontal and vertical, the examiner should not concentrate on the horizontal component at first, since paresis of the vertical muscles may permit a horizontal separation produced by normal esophoria or exophoria.

When the image separation becomes maximal, the examiner knows that the eyes are moving in the direction of action of the weak ocular muscle. Paired or "yoked" ocular muscles are responsible for bringing both eyes conjugately to any given position. For example, the lateral rectus on the right and the medial rectus on the left are responsible for gaze to the right. If diplopia occurs on gaze to the right, it must be due to weakness of one of those two muscles. The examiner's problem is to determine which of the paired muscles is involved. The solution depends on the relative position of the red and white images. The eye with the paretic muscle lags behind in its rotation in the direction of gaze in which diplopia occurs. Because of cortical projection, the image of the paretic eye is seen by the patient to be displaced farthest to the periphery in the direction of gaze. If, in the above instance, with gaze to the right and the red glass over the right eye, the red image is farthest to the patient's right, then there is a paralysis of the right lateral rectus muscle. In another instance, again with the red glass over the right eye, if there is maximal image separation down to the left, and the red image is projected farthest down, paralysis of the right superior oblique muscle can be suspected.

The interpretation of this and all diplopia tests, depends upon the two following cardinal principles:

1. Diplopia (or image separation) increases or worsens as the eye moves in the direction of gaze requiring principally the action of the involved muscle or muscles. (It decreases or disappears in directions of gaze that do not require the action of involved muscle or muscles.)
2. The image seen by the eye with the paretic muscle is displaced farthest to the periphery (*i.e.,* more to the right on right gaze, left on left gaze, higher on upward gaze, lower on downward gaze).

Principle of the Red Glass Test

Figure 6-14 shows that in the normal person both eyes are rotated by the appropriate extraocular muscles so that the image of the flashlight falls on the maculae (M) of both eyes. Figure 6-15 shows the flashlight moved in a lateral direction. Due to adequate rotation of the eyes, the image of the flashlight still falls on both maculae, allowing the brain to superimpose both images into a single image.

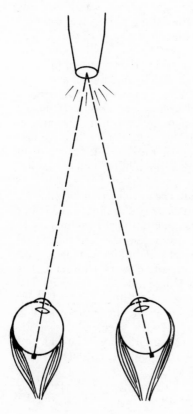

Fig. 6-14. On forward gaze, the image of the light falls on the maculae of both eyes, and one image is seen by the patient because of balanced extraocular activity.

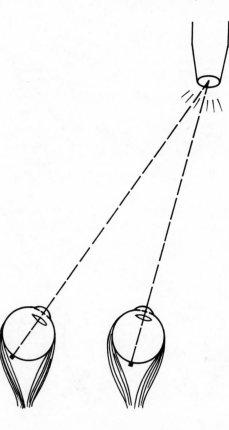

Fig. 6-15. On lateral gaze, one image is still seen as eyes rotate in a manner that ensures that the image falls on both maculae.

Figure 6-16 shows the effect of a weak lateral rectus muscle (indicated by the cross). When the light is moved laterally, the eye with the involved muscle is unable to fully rotate and ensure that the image falls on its macula. As a result, the image falls on the retina medial to the macula, giving the illusion of a laterally displaced image (dotted line), since the medial retina always receives images from the lateral visual field. If one eye had been covered by a red lens, the image for each eye could have been identified by its color so that the eye with the weak muscle could have been identified by its image moving farthest to the periphery.

Opticokinetic Nystagmus

Opticokinetic nystagmus can normally be induced by asking the patient to observe a series of images passing in front of the eyes sideways, from the left and right, up and down. A striped drum, a cloth, or tape measure can be used. The patient is asked to look at each image (stripe, square, number) as it passes in front of his eyes. The produced nystagmus shows a slow component following each passing stimulus (pursuit movement) and a quick jerk as the eyes snap back to catch the next passing stimulus (saccadic or fixation movements). The examiner should note the presence and comparative amplitude of the nystagmus in each direction; the relative presence or absence of both the quick and slow

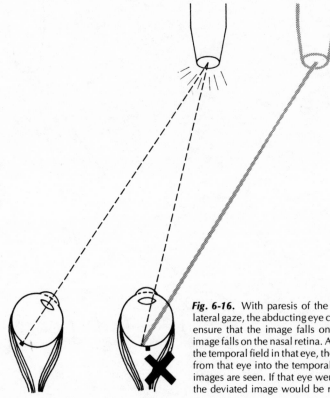

Fig. 6-16. With paresis of the lateral rectus muscle on lateral gaze, the abducting eye cannot move far enough to ensure that the image falls on its macula. Instead, the image falls on the nasal retina. As the nasal retina receives the temporal field in that eye, the brain projects the image from that eye into the temporal field (gray line) and two images are seen. If that eye were covered by a red glass, the deviated image would be red.

component in the nystagmus produced in each direction; and the equality or symmetry of movement in each eye.

Loss of horizontal opticokinetic nystagmus in one direction, coupled with a homonymous hemianopsia, may indicate involvement of the contralateral optic radiations in the parietal lobe. For a more detailed discussion of this valuable test, refer to Glaser's Neurophthalmology (see Bibliography).

CRANIAL NERVE V

Sensation

The tongue (anterior two-thirds), buccal mucosa, gingiva, nasal mucosa, and conjunctiva, are innervated by the trigeminal. All three divisions (ophthalmic, maxillary, mandibular) should be tested, and left and right comparisons should be made. The examiner should know the limits of trigeminal sensation on the face (Fig. 6-17). A pin is the more practical stimulus, but a light tickle touch with a wisp of cotton can be used.

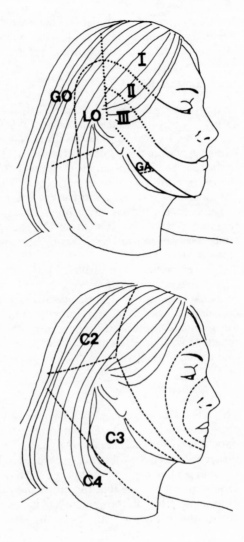

Fig. 6-17. *(A)* Trigeminal peripheral sensory nerve patterns. *I*, ophthalmic division; *II*, maxillary division; *III*, mandibular division; *GA*, greater auricular nerve; *GO*, greater occipital nerve; *LO*, lesser occipital nerve. *(B)* Segmental or "radicular" sensory nerve pattern seen in some intramedullary lesions affecting the trigeminal nucleus and tract. C2, C3 and C4 are the sensory areas of cervical segmental or root patterns.

Muscles of Mastication

The examiner can observe the jaw opening and closing and watch carefully to see if the mentum or lower teeth deviate from the midline. It is important to remember that the jaw deviates to the side of the weak masticator muscles. This would be ipsilateral to the involved fifth nerve or nuclei and contralateral to supranuclear or hemispheric involvement. In patients with acute internal capsule or corticobulbar lesions, the jaw deviates to the contralateral side, but restitution usually occurs in a few days due to ipsilateral corticobulbar innervation. The examiner can also attempt to close the patient's open jaw to see if *resistively?*

deviation occurs. He can palpate the contracting temporalis and masseter muscles during chewing to find evidence of a reduced muscle mass. They can be best palpated at their anterior borders behind the angle of the mouth.

Corneal Reflex

The patient's gaze should be directed upward and laterally to uncover each cornea. The examiner tells the patient that he will be touched on the "white of the eye" with cotton and not to blink. The examiner then touches the patient's sclera away from the cornea and waits for the patient to become accommodated to the touch of the cotton. He then touches the edge of the cornea and observes the reflex blink response in both eyes. With a jumpy or anxious patient, the examiner may have to go to the cornea directly.

The corneal reflex is an early, sensitive, and relatively objective sign of the trigeminal nerve involvement. It is a superficial cutaneous reflex that may be suppressed in contralateral, acute hemispheric lesions affecting the corticospinal tract.

Since the reflex is controlled by the afferent trigeminal and efferent facial nerve bilaterally, the examiner should be careful to determine whether the lack of blink response is due to insensitivity of the cornea or weakness of the obicularis occuli. In an afferent, trigeminal lesion, neither eye will blink when the ipsilateral cornea is touched; both will blink when the contralateral cornea is touched. With an efferent facial nerve lesion, the ipsilateral eye will not blink, and the contralateral eye will blink regardless of the cornea touched.

Jaw Reflex

This reflex arc is probably both afferent and efferent by the motor division of the trigeminal nerve. It is a deep tendon reflex with a reflex center in the pons. In a patient who shows generalized hyperreflexia, the activity of the jaw jerk may differentiate between upper cervical cord or higher brain lesions. If the jaw reflex is not hyperactive, yet all the lower deep tendon reflexes are hyperactive, then the examiner can assume that the upper motor neuron lesion is not as high as the pons bilaterally. If the jaw reflex is hyperactive, then he can assume that corticobulbar involvement above the level of the pons exists bilaterally.

CRANIAL NERVE VII

Again, the examiner should not miss an opportunity to look at the patient's entire face for the characteristic "facies" of myasthenia, myopathy, bulbar paralysis, myotonia dystrophica, hyperthyroidism and Cushing's syndrome.

The frontalis muscles are tested by asking the patient to elevate his eyebrows. The examiner can observe the equality of the forehead furrows or test muscle strength by pulling down on the eyebrows. If the patient finds this difficult, ask him to look far upward or gaze at the finger held above his head, and the frontalis muscle will automatically contract.

The orbicularis oculi can be tested by asking the patient to close his eyes as tightly as possible. With even minimal paresis, the eyelashes can be seen to

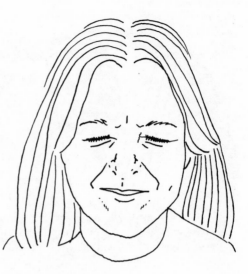

Fig. 6-18. Facial symmetry with forcible eye closure. Note symmetrical nasolabial folds.

protrude farther on the paretic side. The eye may be forced open more easily by the examiner on the paretic side.

Test zygomaticus function by asking the patient to smile or show the teeth. Some people habitually have a wry smile simulating paresis; however, on forced eye closure, they usually show a symmetrical grimace reflexly (Fig. 6-18). With more obvious paresis, the mouth is seen to droop and the nasolabial fold is less prominent on the paretic side. Asking the patient to puff the cheeks and blow through the mouth may also reveal subtle paresis on one side. In addition to a voluntary smile or grimace, the patient should be observed during spontaneous smiling for signs of facial paresis. Observation of the patient's face at rest and during conversation can provide indications of early paresis.

The facial nerve system is helpful in establishing the rostral level of corticospinal involvement. The following guidelines are helpful in considering the locus of damage with facial nerve dysfunction (Fig. 6-19):

1. Peripheral damage to nerve VII
   Here all the muscles on the ipsilateral side are involved to some degree. Taste and lacrimation can be involved, and patients may have hyperacusis ipsilaterally if there are very proximal lesions near the brain stem.
2. Damage to the brain stem and nucleus of nerve VII (pontine)
   This usually looks like a peripheral lesion of nerve VII in that all the muscles on the ipsilateral side are involved. In addition, paresis of the ipsilateral lateral rectus is seen, or an ipsilateral gaze paresis due to involvement of the nerve VI nucleus and lateral gaze center in close proximity to the facial nerve nucleus. There may be contralateral long track signs such as hemiparesis and hemisensory loss.
3. Damage to the central, supranuclear, or upper motor neuron system of nerve VII (corticobulbar system in the internal capsule and cerebral peduncle)
   This is associated with a contralateral facial muscle paresis with sparing of the frontalis muscle due to ipsilateral corticobulbar fibers that also supply the neurons in the facial nerve nucleus that supply this muscle.
4. Cortical supranuclear lesions involving the corticobulbar system of nerve VII

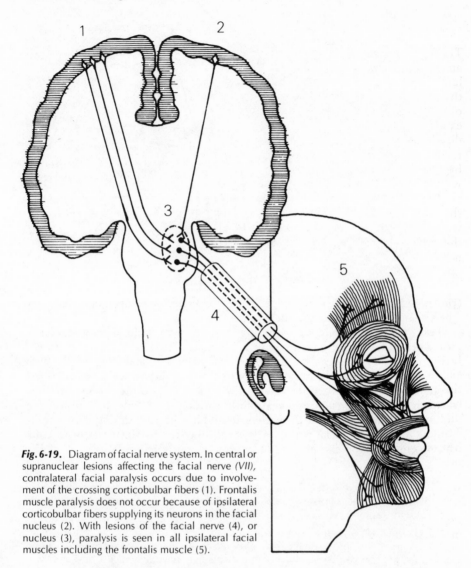

Fig. 6-19. Diagram of facial nerve system. In central or supranuclear lesions affecting the facial nerve *(VII)*, contralateral facial paralysis occurs due to involvement of the crossing corticobulbar fibers (1). Frontalis muscle paralysis does not occur because of ipsilateral corticobulbar fibers supplying its neurons in the facial nucleus (2). With lesions of the facial nerve (4), or nucleus (3), paralysis is seen in all ipsilateral facial muscles including the frontalis muscle (5).

Cortical lesions produce a "voluntary" central facial paresis, identical to the central nerve VII paresis described above (*i.e.,* sparing of the frontalis muscle) seen on voluntary smiling or grimace. However, no paresis is seen on spontaneous smiling or laughter.

5. Deep hemispheric (basal nuclei) lesions involving the upper motor neuron system of nerve VII (mimetic facial paresis)

   These lesions also produce a central type paresis of nerve VII (*i.e.,* sparing of the frontalis muscle) that occurs only on spontaneous smiling or laughter. No paresis is seen on voluntary smiling or grimace.

Taste Test

The nervus intermedius (afferent to the tractus solitarius and gustatory nuclei) is anatomically associated with nerve VII to the chorda tympani near the geniculate ganglion in the inner ear. It is important to evaluate taste (anterior two-thirds of the tongue) in patients with peripheral damage to nerve VII, as absence of taste would indicate such a proximal lesion of nerve VII. For this test, the examiner paints saturated solutions of salt, sugar, vinegar (or citric acid), and diluted quinine solution alternately on each side of the tongue. The tongue must remain outside the mouth while the patient identifies the taste. This can be done by preparing a sheet of paper with the words "sweet, sour, salt, and bitter" written on it. The patient can then identify the taste by pointing to the appropriate word without having to bring his tongue into his mouth to speak. Quinine should be used last since the bitter taste will linger. The patient should drink water between taste substances. A possible difference in lacrimation between the eyes should also be noted in examining for proximal dysfunction of cranial nerve VII.

CRANIAL NERVE VIII

Cochlear Portion of Cranial Nerve VIII

Loss of ability to hear high-frequency tones is characteristic of nerve deafness. In examination of a patient for hearing loss, a high-pitched sound (*e.g.,* lightly ticking watch, light finger rubbing, faint whisper, 2,048 Hz tuning fork) should be used. A low-pitched sound such as a 128 Hz or 256 Hz tuning fork may not disclose neural hearing loss. One ear must be carefully compared to the other. The patient's ears can be compared to the examiner's if the latter is certain his hearing is intact. It is advisable to occlude the ear not being tested by finger pressure on the tragus.

Weber and Rinne Maneuvers When hearing loss is detected, the Weber and Rinne maneuvers should be used to compare air conduction and bone conduction. In the Rinne maneuver, a tuning fork is set in vibration and put on the mastoid process. When the patient says he no longer hears the sound, the fork is put opposite the external auditory meatus. If the patient hears it again, air conduction is greater than bone; if the patient does not hear it, the reverse exists. With higher frequency tuning forks, diminution of sound to inaudible levels may take some time. This can be hastened by putting a finger on the base of the fork and slowly moving up the arm until the sound cannot be heard by the patient.

To perform the Weber maneuver, the vibrating tuning fork is placed on the vertex and the patient is asked where he hears it. If the sound is referred to one side of the head or in one ear (as can be produced by occluding the ear), bone conduction is greater than air conduction on that side. This test is practically useless and often confusing.

Hearing loss with bone conduction greater than air conduction indicates

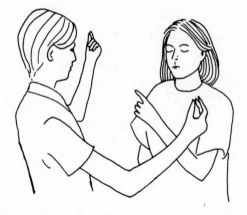

Fig. 6-20. Sound localization in space

nonneurogenic or "conductive" hearing loss indicating such things as occlusion (wax) or involvement of the ossicles in the middle ear (infection, otosclerosis). Hearing loss with air conduction greater than bone conduction indicates neurogenic loss, or so-called "sensorineural" hearing loss.

More clinical information to differentiate end-organ diseases, such as Meniere's disease, from nerve involvement, as in acoustic neuroma or central hearing deficits in brain stem lesions, can be obtained from a large battery of neurootological tests (see p. 116).

Sound Localization in Space The examiner clicks the fingers of the right or left hand in random order and bilaterally simultaneously in different positions around the patient's head. The patient, with eyes closed, is expected to point to the direction of the sound source (Fig. 6-20). Unilateral loss of localization or extinction on bilateral stimuli can suggest a contralateral temporal lobe or subcortical lesion.

Vestibular Portion of Cranial Nerve VIII

Nystagmus Spontaneous nystagmus is usually seen with lesions in the semicircular canals, vestibular nerve, vestibular nuclei and their connections in the brain stem and cerebellum. Nystagmus should be sought in all directions of gaze. The examiner should note the direction of nystagmus (horizontal, vertical, rotary); the presence or absence of the quick component and its direction; the amplitude and speed of nystagmus in each eye and the effect of different directions of gaze; the effects of reclining versus sitting (postural changes); and the duration or persistence of the nystagmus produced by gaze or position change.

The examiner should avoid rotating the patient's neck in these studies, since reflexes from muscle receptors in the neck may affect the quality of postural change on nystagmus or produce a nystagmus.

Test for Veering Veering in walking with the eyes closed, or leaning during the Romberg test, can be seen in patients with unilateral vestibular dysfunction.

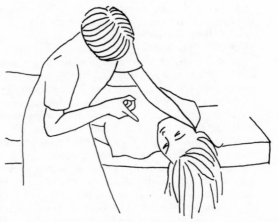

Fig. 6-21. Test for postural vertigo

Marching in Place With a unilateral vestibular lesion, the patient will rotate while marching in place with the eyes closed.

Test for Postural Nystagmus Placed from a sitting position to the dorsal decubitus position with the head extended and rotated over the edge of the bed, the patient is instructed to look straight ahead for approximately one minute (Fig. 6-21). The presence of nystagmus and complaints of vertigo are sought. The test should be repeated with first one ear down and then the other. A sufficient sitting time between tests should be allowed for the patient to recover.

> A positive response to this test points to possible vestibular end-organ involvement as in "benign positional vertigo" or "vestibular neuronitis." An immediate, persistent nystagmus that changes direction with changes in head position, and appears on repeated maneuvers, suggests brain stem or posterior fossa pathology. This is also suspected if the patient shows nystagmus without vertigo. A delayed, mild, rapidly disappearing response that produces a nystagmus in only one direction and cannot be repeated suggests benign postural vertigo. The supine patient can be rolled to one side to effect the same result. As mentioned previously, the examiner should avoid turning the patient's neck.

Test for Past Pointing The patient is first asked to elevate an extended arm over his head with index finger extended. The patient then brings the arm down to touch his index finger to the examiner's outstretched index finger with eyes opened. The test is repeated with the eyes closed. With vestibular system dysfunction, the patient may show drift of the arm preventing accurate placement of the finger. The ball joint of the shoulder is ideal for this test as it allows for lateral motion.

> The vestibular system helps to orient the patient's posture or motor activity to changes in body position. The semicircular canals are arranged on each side in three planes, each containing an endolymph and a cupola that bend with endolymph flow. Rotary or angular acceleration and deceleration affect flow in the endolymph of canals in the plane of rotation. Linear acceleration of the head affects the otolith

organ in the maculae, but the constant effect of gravity makes the sensation of linear movement hard to isolate. This semicircular canal end-organ system is a balanced system. They discharge equally through both nerves VIII to the vestibular nuclei bilaterally. This balanced neural tonus goes to the autonomic nuclei in the brain stem, the nuclei of the extraocular muscles, and the cortex of the cerebrum and cerebellum as well as other brain stem centers. This system allows for compensatory movement of the eyes, limbs, and body when the body is in motion. The system becomes imbalanced when one side discharges more or less than the other. This imbalance can be produced by rotation of the head or douching the external canal with cold or hot water (caloric test) both causing movement of the endolymph and bending of the cupola. If the cupola bends laterally, it increases neural discharges down nerve VIII to the vestibular nucleus, and if it bends medially, the discharge decreases. Imbalance produced by rotation is physiological. Imbalance produced by caloric irrigation is a helpful diagnostic tool as it tests the reactivity of the vestibular system. However, disease or lesions affecting one vestibular system can also produce this imbalance. Since the imbalance can be produced by involvement of the semicircular canals, or nerve VIII, or the vestibular nuclei or their connecting pathways, the examiner must consider carefully the responses produced by the imbalance to locate the patient's problem. The cortical sensation produced by this imbalance is one of rotation, rotation of self or environment—the symptom of vertigo. Reflex changes are produced by this imbalance in the two vestibular systems that are responsible for the signs and symptoms of vestibular disease; nystagmus as the tonus to the paired or "yolked" eye muscles is imbalanced; drift of the arms and legs and deviation of the trunk as descending influences from the brain stem and cerebellum are altered; nausea and vomiting from reflex connections in the medulla affecting peristalsis. The presence of all these responses when the patient's body is still suggests end-organ or nerve VIII disease. By contrast, central lesions of the vestibular system or its pathways tend to cause only part of these responses to occur.

Possible Symptoms of Central or Brain Stem Lesions

Nystagmus without vertigo

Nystagmus and vertigo without nausea

Vertigo and nausea without nystagmus

Change of nystagmus direction on change of posture or change of gaze (unless drug-induced)

Dissociated or distorted nystagmus (i.e., vertical in one eye and horizontal in the other, nystagmus greater in one side than the other, tonic adduction of one eye and nystagmus in the other)

Nonfatiguing nystagmus on posture change

Vertical nystagmus (unless drug-induced)

Nystagmus caused by end-organ or peripheral nerve lesions tends to disappear after three weeks; persistence supports the likelihood of central damage. Evidence of hearing loss or auditory symptoms also suggests a peripheral cause. It is helpful to remember a generalization that the slow component of the nystagmus, the drift of the arms and trunk, the veering of the gait tends toward the side of vestibular nerve or end-organ damage or the side away from a warm caloric stimulus or toward a cold caloric stimulus.

False nystagmus due to competition between convergence and lateral gaze on far extremes of gaze can be minimized if the examiner holds his finger farther from the patient's eyes to lessen convergence. Nystagmus can be seen in patients with minimal neuromuscular weakness of the extraocular muscles.

A large battery of neurootological tests are available to better determine whether the vestibular signs are of peripheral or central origin, and, if peripheral, whether they are due to end-organ involvement or involvement of the peripheral nerve (retrochlear). For further information see Clinical Neurophysiology of the Vestibular System by Baloh and Honrubia (see Bibliography).

The examiner must attempt to determine where the vestibular damage is located (end-organ, peripheral nerve, brain stem, hemisphere).

CRANIAL NERVES IX—X

These cranial nerves are clinically inseparable. The activities of the vagus nerve on cardiac, respiratory, and gastrointestinal function are difficult to assay because of the variable suprasegmental and hormonal influences on the autonomic system. The neurologic examination is usually limited to evaluation of sensation in the posterior oral cavity and pharynx, pharyngeal and vocal muscles, and the gag reflex.

Palate Movement

Equal movement of left and right palate is sought on vocalization or stimulation by gag. The uvula will be seen to deviate away from the side of palatal paresis. The bilateral symmetrical contractions of the stylopharyngeous muscles may be a more reliable guide if the soft palate has been fibrosed secondary to tonsillectomy on one side, causing the uvula to deviate to the side of the scar.

Tracheal Movement

The examiner watches the patient swallow water in order to observe the tracheal movement and its adequacy.

Gag Reflex and Sensory Testing

The examiner touches each side of the patient's posterior pharyngeal wall to compare the right and left gag reflex (afferent, efferent IX and X nerves); sensation on both sides of the pharynx can be estimated by asking the patient if the stimulus used in eliciting the gag reflex feels the same on both sides.

The system of cranial nerves IX and X can be further tested by observing the vocal cords with indirect laryngoscopy. This is important when the patient has a history of a change of voice or if a change is noticed on examination. The examiner can also observe the patient's ability to swallow rapidly and note if there is fatigue on continued swallowing, as may be seen in patients with myasthenia gravis. Nasal regurgitation on rapid swallowing can indicate weakness of the soft palate bilaterally. The examiner can also ask the patient to puff his cheeks full of air. Leakage through the nose makes this performance difficult if there is weakness in the muscles of the soft palate. The leakage can be stopped by pinching the patient's nose.

The examiner should remember that the corticobulbar influence on these nuclei is bilateral. Therefore, (1) unilateral deficits of these functions indicate cranial nerve or brain stem nuclear damage ipsilaterally (decreased movements, decreased sensation, decreased gag); (2) bilateral involvement of motor function can be due to bilateral brain stem, cranial nerve, or bilateral corticobulbar damage in the cerebrum. (The syndrome of true bulbar and "pseudobulbar" palsy is described under Cranial Nerve XII).

CRANIAL NERVE XI

The examiner tests sternocleidomastoid function by resisting the patient's head-turning movement. The muscle is observed and palpated; the left sternocleidomastoid muscle turns the head to the right and vice versa. The upper trapezius muscle is tested by asking the patient to elevate the shoulders bilaterally. Both sets of muscles are normally quite strong.

The nuclei of nerve XI, nerve XI itself, and corticospinal system all supply the ipsilateral sternocleidomastoid muscle. In severe internal capsule damage, the patient's head is turned away from the hemiplegic side because the contralateral extremity muscles and the ipsilateral sternocleidomastoid are paralyzed.

CRANIAL NERVE XII

Inspection of the Tongue

The examiner should note the appearance of the tongue at rest in the open mouth and palpate the protruding tongue for evidence of atrophy. Atrophy is usually seen first on the margins and appears as a chipping away. Atrophy is almost always associated with fibrillations.

Protrusion of the Tongue When protruded, the tongue will deviate to the side of the weak muscles if there is unilateral weakness. Therefore, tongue deviation goes to the side of lower motor neuron weakness and opposite the side of upper motor neuron weakness.

In patients with facial paresis, the protruding tongue can appear to deviate to one side. However, if the tongue is protruding straight, the median raphe of the tongue is in line with the tip of the nose and the tip of the chin.

Strength of tongue deviation to each side can be compared by having the patient push against the examiner's finger through a cheek or push a tongue blade to the side. The examiner can also observe the patient's ability to laterally deviate the tongue.

Wiggling of the Tongue The speed and adroitness of wiggling can be affected by parkinsonism, supranuclear palsy, and bulbar palsy (bilateral involvement).

Skills of Articulation With bilateral nuclear, nerve, or corticobulbar dysfunction, no matter how minimal, the patient can evidence dysarthria. Signs of minimal dysarthria can be elicited by having the patient say such catch phrases as "methodist episcopal," "newly laid linoleum," or rapidly repeat "la-la-la-la-la-la." It is important to be sure that lingual sounds are being tested and not labial sounds, which are produced by the lips or the system of nerve VII. Labial movements form such words as "paper bag."

Although the hypoglossal nuclei receive bilateral corticobulbar innervation, acute internal capsule lesions can show contralateral deviation of the tongue initially. Restitution usually occurs in a few days as ipsilateral corticobulbar control takes over. Fibrillation, atrophy, or unilateral paresis usually indicate ipsilateral brain stem, nuclear, or nerve dysfunction. Bilateral involvement of the tongue can be seen in either true bulbar or pseudobulbar palsy.

PSEUDOBULBAR PALSY

Pseudobulbar palsy is seen in patients with bilateral corticobulbar lesions. It can be seen with lesions too slight to show obvious paresis in the face or extremities. Bilateral minimal corticobulbar lesions seem to noticeably affect those cranial nerves with bilateral corticobulbar supply involving articulation and swallowing. In the patient with a hemiparesis or even minimal evidence of paralysis who has, in addition, difficulty in swallowing and articulating, bilateral damage in the nervous system should be suspected. With the pseudobulbar syndrome, the involvement of the corticobulbar system may be anywhere from the cortex bilaterally down through the medulla bilaterally. In the pseudobulbar syndrome, the patient also may show emotional incontinence in that he may laugh but will usually cry with excessive grimacing and with little control. This response is usually triggered by minimally humorous or sad situations. The patients usually have bilateral extensor plantar reflexes, an increased jaw jerk, and often hyperactive gag reflexes. A characteristic short step gait may be seen.

TRUE BULBAR PALSY

True bulbar palsy is seen with bilateral brain stem lesions affecting the cranial nerve nuclei or peripheral nerves involved in swallowing and articulation. It may be differentiated from pseudobulbar palsy by the presence of atrophy or fibrillation of the tongue, sensory loss in the pharyngeal paresis, decreased gag reflex and other lower motor neuron cranial deficits, if present.

TYPES OF DYSARTHRIA

The dysarthria of pseudobulbar involvement (spastic dysarthria) is slow and monotonous with severe impairment of consonants, which sound strained or strangled. The dysarthria of true bulbar palsy is strikingly nasal in quality, short and breathless; the patient is often described as sounding as if a "hot potato" were in his mouth. The dysarthria of cerebellar disease has been coined "scanning speech" because of the unusual stress placed on usually unstressed syllables and words, causing the prosody of speech to be almost singsong in quality. The speech is slow with prolonged sounds. The dysarthria of extrapyramidal disease is revealed in the quiet, short, stressless, monotonous speech of patients with parkinsonism or the explosive, irregular, interrupted, distorted speech of patients with the dyskinesias.

7

MENINGES, PERIPHERAL NERVES, VESSELS, AND BONES

The following group of tests are an intimate part of the neurological examination, but are difficult to classify under any particular system.

MANEUVER FOR NUCHAL RIGIDITY

In meningitis or meningeal inflammation due either to infection of the meninges or to chemical irritation, as in subarachnoid hemorrhage, resistance may be felt on attempted passive flexion of the patient's neck. The examiner can estimate the degree of nuchal rigidity by observing how closely the point of the patient's chin is able to approximate the sternum (Fig. 7-1). Since cervical osteoarthritis may restrict neck flexion in the older patient, it is important to passively rotate the patient's head laterally prior to testing for nuchal rigidity. In cervical osteoarthritis, lateral rotation of the head causes resistance as well as forward flexion. In meningeal irritation, lateral rotation of the head is uninvolved. On forward flexion, the patient with meningitis usually feels pain down the back or neck and exacerbation of any headache that might be present (see the discussion of neck examination, p. 126).

MANEUVERS FOR ROOT OR MENINGEAL IRRITATION

These maneuvers are often labelled with a series of eponyms, some incorrectly applied. It is probably wise to forget the eponyms.

One method is to see how far the knee can be extended after the thigh has been fully flexed (Fig. 7-2). Most people have difficulty with full knee extension in this position; discomfort and pulling are felt in the popliteal space. Meningeal or root irritation will cause resistance to knee extension and/or pain along the path of the sciatic nerve into the buttock and back.

Another maneuver is the passive elevation of a leg with the knee extended (Fig. 7-3). The examiner makes sure that the patient keeps the pelvis flat on the surface of the examining table by putting a restraining hand on the pelvis. Again,

120

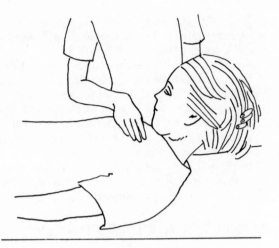

Fig. 7-1. Test for nuchal rigidity

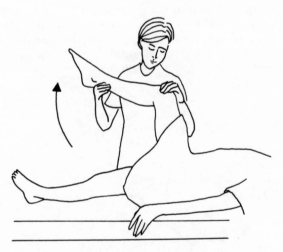

Fig. 7-2. Extending the knee with
the hip flexed

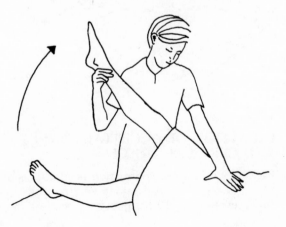

Fig. 7-3. Flexing the hip with the
knee extended

meningeal irritation or root involvement will cause pain and resistance to straight leg raising. The examiner should note to what degree of angle from the bed the patient is able to tolerate flexion of the extended leg at the hips.

A confirmatory test in these maneuvers is forcible, passive dorsiflexion of the patient's ankle while the straight leg is flexed at the hip as far as tolerated. This produces an additional pull on the nerve roots and meninges, further aggravating the patient's back in pain of meningeal or sciatic origin.

With meningitis, other signs may be seen, such as the inability of the patient to flex forward in sitting. This movement often requires placement of the arms behind to maintain the sitting posture (tripod stance).

In the patient with meningitis, forcible flexion of the neck causes a reflex flexion of both knees. This confirmatory test should be reserved for the severely obtunded or comatose patient since it can be very painful.

MANEUVER FOR HIP PATHOLOGY

Since disease of the hip may simulate meningeal or nerve root irritation by causing pain during the above maneuvers, it is important for the examiner to flex the patient's knee, place the foot on the contralateral knee and externally rotate the thigh until it is nearly flat on the table (Fig. 7-4). This maneuver is not tolerated in patients with hip disease, but it produces no discomfort in those with root or meningeal irritation.

> These tests assay involvement of the nerve roots from approximately L4 and below. To test for nerve root irritation at the L3 to L4 level, the patient's hip should be hyperextended since these roots lie above the ascetabulum and would not be stretched by hip flexion.

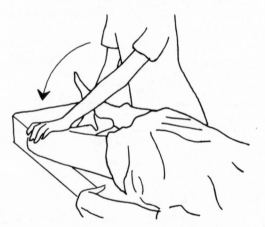

Fig. 7-4. A test to rule out hip pathology

PALPATION OF OCCIPITAL NERVES AND CERVICAL MUSCLES

Patients with muscle contraction headaches, posterior fossa mass lesions, or high cervical spinal cord lesions will frequently have headaches and occipital or suboccipital pain. Palpation of the exit of the occipital nerves may reveal tenderness, and may often aggravate or reproduce the pain or headache. The points of exit are behind the mastoid process and in the suboccipital notch. In addition, palpation of the posterior neck muscles may reveal spasm and tenderness. Palpation of the suboccipital articulation and cervical spinous processes should also be performed. Spasm of the posterior cervical muscles and trapezius is best felt with the patient fully relaxed in the dorsal decubitus position without a pillow.

EXAMINATION AND PALPATION OF SCALP

Careful examination may be difficult on the patient with abundant hair, but inspection for evidence of tumors or bumps, abnormal markings or vessels, skull symmetry, depressed skull fractures, old craniotomy sites, can be helpful. The temporal artery should be palpated for indication of tenderness with suspected temporal arteritis.

NERVE TENDERNESS

Tenderness of the brachial plexus can be elicited by stretching the patient's arm. Tenderness of the nerves in the lumbar plexus can be produced by leg maneuvers described above. Tenderness of the nerves in the arm and leg can be elicited by direct compression over the nerves. This is done most conveniently on the medial side of the arm and in the posterior aspect of the calf. It is important to differentiate muscle tenderness from nerve tenderness. Muscle tenderness is felt to exist if lateral compression of the muscles of the arm or the leg produces more tenderness to the patient than compression directly over the nerve trunk. For example, lateral compression of the calf muscle should be compared to compression over the posterior surface of the calf muscle. If lateral compression of the calf muscle is more tender, the examiner can assume muscle tenderness is present. If posterior tenderness is greater, nerve tenderness is present.

Tinel's Sign

The sign refers to tingling dysesthesias produced by percussion over the area of regeneration of a damaged peripheral nerve.

THORACOCERVICAL ROOT OUTLET MANEUVERS

A variety of lesions can involve the brachial plexus and the vascular supply to the arm since these structures pass through the strap muscles in the neck between the clavicle and first rib, and under the pectoralis minor tendon. These structures are important in evaluation of pain, tingling, weakness, and sensory loss in the arms. Several maneuvers are used to elicit evidence of compression of the nerves or vessels in this thoracocervical outlet. In these maneuvers, if the patient complains of pain, numbness, or tingling in the fingers, compression of nerves is assumed. In addition, the examiner has his fingers on the radial pulse, and if the

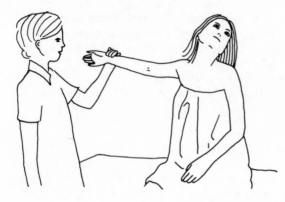

Fig. 7-5. Thoracocervical root outlet maneuver: full rotation of the head with the neck extended

pulse disappears during these maneuvers, then he can assume that vascular compression has occurred. This latter can be verified by sphygmomanometer or oscillometer readings, and by hearing bruit in the supraclavicular or subclavicular space during these maneuvers.

The examiner holds the patient's arm out laterally and asks the patient to extend his head then turn his head to the far extremes of lateral motion (Fig. 7-5). The examiner then elevates the patient's arms high over the head. Even in some normal patients, the pulse will be felt to diminish bilaterally with this maneuver. Next, the patient is instructed to hyperabduct the shoulders. If this produces no symptoms or pulse deficit, then the patient is asked to perform a Valsalva maneuver. Finally, the examiner presses the patient's shoulder forcibly downward, stretching the neurovascular bundle.

Anomalies (*e.g.*, cervical ribs, old fractures of the clavicle with callus formation, and ptosis of the shoulder girdle) can be responsible for a variety of pain and sensory syndromes in the arm. In some women, hyperabduction of the shoulders will depress the pulse in both wrists; this finding is of no clinical significance.

PERIPHERAL NERVE PALPATION

Palpation of peripheral nerves may disclose atrophy, enlargement (hypothyroidism, interstitial hypertrophy), increased tenderness or total insensitivity, all of which can be important in assessing the patient's particular peripheral nerve problem.

Ulnar Nerve

The ulnar nerve can be felt just proximal to the notch on the dorsal surface of the medial malleolus of the humerus (Fig. 7-6).

Peroneal Nerve

The peroneal nerve can be felt distal to the head of the fibula as it sweeps across the shaft of the fibula (Fig. 7-7).

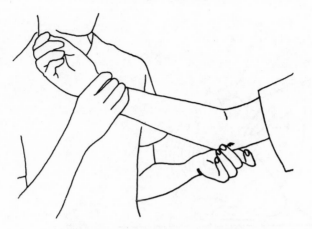

Fig. 7-6. Palpation of the ulnar nerve

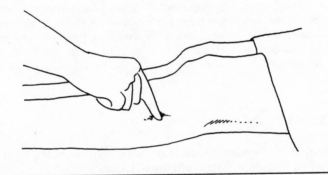

Fig. 7-7. Palpation of the peroneal nerve

PALPATION OF ARTERIES

Although palpation of the major arteries is part of the routine physical examination, it is especially important during the neurological examination to carefully palpate the carotid arteries to search for inequality of pulsation, bruit, or absence of pulsation. The optimal position for this examination is with the patient recumbent and the head slightly extended (Fig. 7-8).

The radial and pedal arteries should also be palpated routinely in the neurological examination. The temporal arteries should be palpated for induration, and especially for enlargement or tenderness in patients with suspected temporal arteritis.

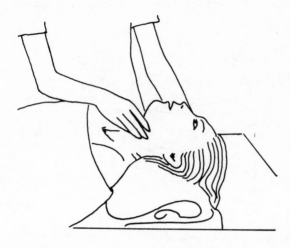

Fig. 7-8. Palpation of the carotid arteries

AUSCULATION OF ARTERIES

Ausculation of the carotids for murmurs, bruit, or reduced sound may disclose extracranial vascular disease. It is important for the examiner to note whether the sounds he hears are conducted from the heart or originate in the carotids themselves. Auscultation of the subclavian, brachial, and axillary arteries can be of value in evaluation of vascular disease or root outlet syndromes. It is also possible on occasions to hear bruit over the vertebral arteries in the posterior neck.

NECK EXAMINATION

The range of motion, flexion, extension (anteroposterior, right-left), and rotation should be examined through both active and passive motion to see if there is restricted mobility due to arthritis, cervical disc disease, or muscle spasm. The cervical muscles should be examined and palpated for evidence of tenderness or spasm. In patients with suspected lateral intervertebral disc protrusion, the pain can be aggravated by pressing down on the head with the neck flexed toward the painful side. Traction of the neck, by elevating the head, may relieve the pain.

AUSCULTATION OF THE HEAD

Vascular malformations and aneurysms may, on rare occasions, produce audible bruit in the head. The head should be auscultated over the orbits, and in the frontal, parietal, and occipital areas. The orbital areas are particularly advantageous in that access to sounds within the skull is improved. To avoid noise interference created by the orbicularis oculi, the patient should be instructed to open the eye on the side that is not being auscultated.

8

MENTAL STATUS
(Including Communication Skills)

The human cortex is often described as having areas that relate to specific functions. There are primary sensory areas in the anterior portions of the parietal cortex (touch), medial occipital cortex (vision), and superior temporal cortex (hearing). Primary motor areas are in the frontal cortex. The so-called limbic system occupies a long circular band of the cortex on the medial surface of the hemispheres and is involved in emotional responses, memory, and the autonomic component of emotional activity. The term "associative cortex" refers to those large cortical areas that lie between the primary motor and sensory areas, and are important to all varieties of communication skills in the human. These functional categories are a convenience to the clinician in analyzing the symptoms and signs of cortical lesions but should not imply that the cortex is a mosaic of isolated functions. The remainder of the cortex, frontal and temporal, provides the human with unique capacities often referred to as "highest integrative functions of the brain." Along with such terms as "memory, thought, and emotion," these functions are also encompassed by such semantically loaded concepts as "mind, character, personality, and intelligence." It is these qualities of human performance that are affected by disease processes that involve the cortex diffusely or in multiple areas. The clinical syndromes presented by such disorders have been labelled with such terms as "organic brain syndrome" and "dementia." The clinician, in his examination, tends to look for more easily measurable signs of generalized cortical dysfunction (*e.g.,* orientation, memory, calculation, fund of general information, judgment, adaptability).

The mental mechanisms used by humans to adapt life-style, conflicts, and environmental adversities into socially acceptable behavior must also be an overall function of the cortex. Patients with an organic brain syndrome may have bizarre or psychotic behavior which, on investigation, can usually be found to represent an exaggeration of their premorbid personality pattern. This data is best elicited by inquiry of close acquaintances or family. The contributions of the limbic system and its connections with the hypothalamus and diencephalon to the organic brain syndrome may be seen in disorders of emotional tone (*e.g.,* toxic or metabolic derangements manifested by delirium, agitation, combative-ness, hallucinations, delusions, withdrawal).

Bilateral frontal lobe pathology alone can produce many of the objective manifestations of organic brain syndrome since the frontal lobes represent a large portion of cortex and possess rich connections to limbic lobe and temporal lobe systems. In assaying the patient's mental status, the examiner should be aware of (1) the patient's level of formal education, (2) the patient's level of consciousness, and (3) the patient's ability to communicate.

TESTS FOR MENTAL STATUS

Orientation

To test the patient's orientation to place, the examiner determines the patient's knowledge of where he is located in both large term (*e.g.*, city and state) and small details (*e.g.*, the building he is in and its specific location).

Orientation to time is tested by asking the patient about the time of day, day of the week, month, and year.

Orientation to person is rarely lost even in patients with the most severe organic brain disease. Such loss is more often a manifestation of psychosis.

Memory

To test for recent recall, the examiner can interrogate the patient about current events, or he can give the patient an address to remember and ask him to repeat it five or ten minutes later. History taking will elicit a good deal of information in this area. More immediate recall can be tested by having the patient repeat a series of numbers forward or backward.

To test for past memory, the examiner can ask about significant dates in history and events in the patient's lifetime, such as birthdays and wedding dates.

Calculation

A routine screening for calculation can be accomplished by asking the patient to subtract 7 from 100 and continue on in a serial order. This tests not only calculation, but also attention span and immediate recall. After the patient finishes the series successfully, he can then be asked if the remainder is proper and if he knows any arithmetical short cuts for checking it. Further tests for calculation can be made up by the examiner as an appropriate challenge to the particular patient.

Information

The patient's level of factual information can be estimated by asking him about current news events or items of common knowledge in his environment or occupation. Ideas for such questions can be gotten from formal intelligence tests. Everyone should know such things as details about national flags, names and locations of large cities, simple facts about the physics of shadows and movements of the sun. Questions from various intelligence tests can be used by the examiner if he wishes a more measurable result.

Judgment

Judgment can be best estimated by presenting the patient with a problem story which requires a decision, solution, or detection of an absurdity; ideas for testing of judgment can be found in any formal intelligence test. The following is an example: "Railroad companies were concerned about the loss of life and limb in railroad accidents. Investigation shows that the majority of persons killed or injured in a train wreck were in the last car. As a safety precaution, it was recommended that the last car on every train be removed."

Abstract Thinking

This cognitive skill is estimated by asking the patient the meaning of such common proverbs as, "A rolling stone gathers no moss," or "The emptiest drum makes the loudest noise." The examiner notes whether the patient used abstract thought in his answers or was concrete in his thinking. The latter is an early sign of organic brain damage. Examples of concrete thought would be the statement, "If a stone moves constantly, it is impossible for moss to root on it," or "The emptiest drum is capable of a greater amplitude of vibration and, therefore, produces a louder noise." The more severely damaged patient may not understand the proverb. The examiner must be certain that any proverbs and idiomatic sayings used are familiar to the patient and part of his culture and background.

Insight

The examiner should determine whether the patient understands why he is being seen. Does the patient recognize the severity and extent of his disability or illness? Does he appreciate the effect of these difficulties on his future?

During the mental status tests, the examiner should look for other evidence of disordered mental performance (*e.g.*, hallucinations, paranoid thinking, agitation, or depressed motor activity, abnormalities in facial appearance or stream of talk).

EXAMINATION OF COMMUNICATION SKILLS (APHASIA TESTING)

Disordered function in the associative cortex of the dominant hemisphere for language is usually expressed as a loss of communication skills. This cortex, located between the frontal, temporal, parietal and occipital cortices, plays a crucial role in integrating past and present sensory data into an effective motor pattern for expression in locomotion, speech, writing, and gestures.

There are three primary modes of input for human communication: audition, vision, and tactile sensation. The other senses play a minor role in communication. There are also three modes of output in communication: speech, graphic skills (writing, drawing), and kinetic skills (gestures, facial expressions, pantomime). In communication with other people, the patient receives information from one of the input modes and transmits responses, reactions, ideas, or concepts through one of the outputs (Fig. 8-1).

Recognition of these three inputs and outputs provides a structure for examining the patient with a communication disorder. It allows the examiner to fully explore the patient's ability to communicate. It also makes the examiner aware of the fact that a single manifestation of disordered communication can have multiple causes. He must be careful not to incorrectly identify which disordered function is responsible for the communication disorder the patient shows. For example, if the patient cannot name an object shown to him, the examiner must determine whether this is due to a lack of recognition, an inability to recall, or an inability to enunciate the object's name.

The response of the individual's disordered cortex is not only exceedingly complex, but probably unique to the personality of the patient affected. The actual patterns of association in each individual are as unique as fingerprints or facial characteristics, and are a product of inheritance, past experiences, and learning style.

The examination should take place in a quiet area free from distracting noise. The examiner should speak clearly and slowly, repeating as often as necessary. He must have allocated sufficient time to perform this examination so that he does not communicate pressure or a sense of hurry to the patient. The examiner should present each test item singly to the patient and should not allow test items and materials to clutter the area around the patient, providing distracting stimuli. If the patient shows evidence of fatigue, the examiner should stop and continue at another time.

The examiner should also be aware of the following factors that may coexist with a communication disorder and interfere with communication:

1. Perseveration is a response to one command that is subsequently given as a response to all following commands even though they may be of a different nature. For example, if the patient is asked to close his eyes, and then subsequently asked to stick out his tongue or raise his arm, he will continue to close his eyes. If perseveration continues to become more frequent and severe, the examiner should stop and continue the examination at another time or another day since it can inhibit all communication. Perseveration can suggest involvement of the frontal lobe.

2. Confabulation is an amnesic syndrome in which the patient fills in a loss of recent memory with fantasies or events that never occurred. In addition, patients with this syndrome may have an inability to acquire new learning or recent memories. This is the central element in the so-called Korsakoff's psychosis and frequently accompanies alcoholism. However, it is important for the examiner to realize that confabulation can occur with hemispheric disease and can confound communication to a marked degree. This can suggest involvement of the limbic lobe or mesial temporal lobe.

3. Associated psychological deficits may be exhibited along with communication disorders. The patient may appear confused, may be very inattentive, show emotional instability and unfavorable psychological attitudes to his disability (*e.g.,* fatigue, depression, discouragement, intolerance to the interview situation). Recognition of these problems is important so that the examiner will

INPUT (reception)   OUTPUT (expression)

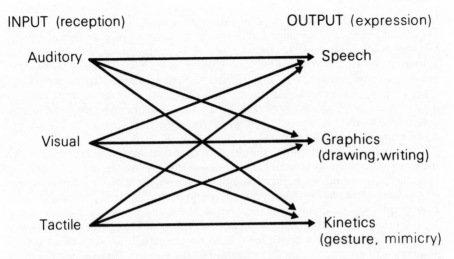

Fig.8-1. Communication schema. Adapted from Monrad-Krohn, G. H., The Clinical Examination of the Nervous System, p. 271, P. B. Hoeber Inc., New York, 1955.

modify his approach to compensate for these problems in the patient. They also indicate more diffuse cortical involvement than may be suggested by the communication disorder alone. It is important that the examiner show no signs of reaction to the patient's difficulty that might suggest pity, humor, or repulsion. These demonstrations only engender negative responses from the patient and inhibit communication.

It is probably a mistake for the examiner to feel that the communication can provide him with a precise localization of cerebral pathology. It is safe enough to assume that a communication disorder implies a lesion in the cerebral cortex or immediate subadjacent white matter. As to specific areas or loci within the hemisphere, most communication disorders are less specific. Probably the most effective method of localization the examiner can use is to determine first that a communication disorder does exist; it follows that the patient has a disorder of the associative cortex in the so-called "dominant" hemisphere for language. In the great majority of individuals, it will be the left hemisphere. In a few left-handed individuals, it may be the right hemisphere, but this is rare. Secondly, the patient's communication disorder may indicate that the lesion is anterior to the central sulcus (precentral) or posterior to the central sulcus (postcentral). The following is a suggested routine for the bedside evaluation of communication disorder filled in by approaches suggested by Figure 8-1.

Informal Conversation

The examiner should first engage the patient in a relaxed and informal conversation; the patient should not be aware of being tested. During this informal conversation, it is important that the examiner evaluate the characteristic of the patient's speech. The first characteristic of importance is the rate of fluency of the speech. Fluency is a function of rate and speech facility. Is the speech hesitant?

Does it require effort on the part of the patient? Is there perseveration? Are there associated grunts and groans? These would indicate a precentral localization. Overproductive, tangential, rambling speech is characteristic of a postcentral sulcus disorder. It is remarkable how patients who have difficulty in fluency, pointing to a precentral disorder, will have facility with automatic or emotional speech. They may respond with "good morning," swear at appropriate stimuli, or say a number of automatic phrases which are not deliberately and voluntarily determined by the patient. In fact, this may fool the examiner into feeling there is no communication disorder.

The next item the examiner should note in the informal conversation is the presence of word substitutions, the coining of new words, or unintelligible speech. These are more characteristic of lesions posterior to the central sulcus. The grammatical features of the speech should be noted. If the patient speaks in a telegraphic style utilizing primarily nouns, verbs, and pronouns, a communication disorder associated with a precentral lesion is implied. If the patient's speech is hyperfluent, a postcentral lesion is indicated. Lastly, the examiner should be aware of the effective response of the patient. If the patient is quite aware of his communication disorder, showing irritation at his inability to produce the necessary words, or continually hesitates and rephrases or repeats in an attempt to produce more accurate speech, a precentral lesion is suggested. However, if the patient rambles on and is absolutely oblivious of his difficulties, a postcentral lesion is implied.

Comprehension of Spoken Language

To assess the patient's comprehension of spoken language, the examiner can give him a series of commands or instructions that are graded in their complexity. As mentioned before, intact performance indicates a considerable facility in communication, but a poor performance in following commands may be due to a multitude of causes. Another method is to present the patient with a collection of common objects (*e.g.,* paper clips, pencils, pens, coins, pins) and ask the patient to either point to them or pick them up and put them in a cup, or pick them up and perform some sort of activity with them. It is important to realize verbal memory is implied in the performance of more complex tasks. Comprehension can be further challenged by giving the patient contingent instruction. In such instruction, the examiner asks the patient to produce a certain type of response following a performance by the examiner. For example, the examiner may say, "When I raise my hand, you pick up the pen and place it in the cup." Poor comprehension usually points to postcentral disorder.

Repetition

The examiner asks the patient to repeat after him the names of letters, numbers, words, sentences, and various tongue twisters. It is important that he listen carefully for evidence of dysarthria. If the patient is not fluent, an anterior lesion may exist. Ask the patient to recite a series, such as the days of the week or the months of the year. Often poorly fluent patients, if started, will go on through the end of the series with considerable and surprising fluency. Along this line, it is sometimes valuable to see if the patient can sing. Patients with anterior lesions and poor fluency may show an amazing ability to sing verse after verse of songs so long as the words are associated with the melody. Repetition ability should be estimated for both long words and complex phrases, as well as for short phrases with small words, such as, "no ifs, ands, or buts."

Naming Objects

This is a sensitive test of communication function. The examiner shows a number of objects to the patient and asks their names. If the patient is not able to name the object, it is important for the examiner to ascertain whether this is because the patient cannot provide the name or does not recognize the object. If the patient can demonstrate the use of the object (*e.g.,* twisting a key as if in a lock, or opening and making writing movements with a pen), then the examiner can safely assume he recognizes the object but cannot provide its name. Another method is to show a series of objects, as before, and ask the patient to select one. This implies recognition of the object. The lack of facility in word selection is a very sensitive indicator of communication disorder, but does not imply anterior or posterior location, since either may be the case. The examiner can only assume that the associative cortex is involved.

Comprehension of Written Material

In this test, the patient is asked to read words or commands that have been written by the examiner. The patient may either describe the word verbally, or, if he is unable to do this, he may execute a written command, such as, "close your eyes," or "stick out your tongue." Another method to nonverbally test comprehension is to use a series of words written on individual cards and a series of illustrations of those words on another set of cards. The patient is asked to match them.

Writing

Spontaneous writing is the best test. As in speech, the examiner looks for grammatical errors and errors of syntax. He can ask the patient to follow dictation from simple to complex material, and he can ask the patient to copy words or sentences. It is important to make a distinction between signs of paralysis and praxic disorders.

Drawing

Disorders of drawing have been covered previously in the sensory examination and in the examination of visual fields. However, if the patient's drawing shows inattention to one half of the page, a "minor" (right) hemisphere lesion in the parietal cortex or a homonymous hemianopsia is implied. Formal examination should be able to distinguish between these two. If the drawing is very primitive or simplified, a "dominant" hemisphere lesion is suggested.

Spatial Orientation

This is a specialized aspect of cerebral function and cannot be easily classified under communication. However, patients with communication disorders frequently show problems in orientation, either left-right orientation or orientation in space. This type of disorientation can be seen with lesions in the hemisphere opposite the one for language (right). Topographic location, best evaluated by watching the patient move around the room or on the ward from bathroom to bed, can be a sensitive index of general cerebral function; it is severely impaired in the confused patient. The partially comatose or demented patient cannot be successfully examined for a communication disorder. The patient must be aware of his environment and the examiner's activities before a communication disorder can be tested. Therefore, the level of consciousness should be determined. In the severely demented patient, it is of little consequence to identify the communication disorder since this is but one aspect of severe generalized cortical dysfunction.

Summary

In the mental status examination, the examiner should be able to decide: (1) whether a communication disorder is present; (2) which hemisphere is implicated, by noting patient's handedness and other deficits in sensation, motor performance, vision, or reflexes that may point to the involved hemisphere; (3) whether the lesion is focal, multiple, or diffuse by noting other deficits (*e.g.*, confusion, memory loss, bilateral neurological signs), (4) whether there are clear deficits in input or output that may more accurately locate the associative cortex lesion as being nearer the occipital, parietal, temporal, or frontal lobe.

It is important to put the signs of communication deficit together with findings from the rest of the neurological examination, particularly those that reflect cortical or subcortical function (e.g., apraxias, hemiparesis, increased reflexes or tone, extensor plantar responses, hemisensory loss, asterognosis, parietal lobe sensory deficits, homonymous visual field deficits, and mental status).

There is a rare but important group of communication deficits that suggest involvement of interhemispheric connections (e.g., the corpus callosum that carries information from the opposite, nonlanguage hemisphere to the associative cortex of the hemisphere for language). A discussion of these deficits seems inappropriate here, but can be found in the works of Geschwind (see Bibliography).

The language examination and analyses performed by speech therapists are far more extensive than those usually performed by the neurologist. They employ a terminology and classification aimed less at locating the area of cortical deficit, the concern of the neurologist, but more at surveying the patient's total assets and deficits in a manner that will indicate appropriate therapy and treatment. This is no different from the contrast between the motor assessment of the physiotherapist and that of the neurologist, again due to different tasks and goals in the care of the patient.

In the field of neurology, there is a group of specialists who subscribe to a classification of communication disorder syndromes that has an impressive historical perspective of research spanning many decades. An oversimplified version of this classification is given below.

1. Global aphasia: widespread involvement of the language associative cortex. The patient is not fluent, shows no speech comprehension, cannot repeat, and makes

stereotyped utterances that can show emotional inflection. This aphasia usually clears in a few days and assumes the characteristics of a Broca's aphasia.

2. Broca's (expressive, motor) aphasia: involvement of the speech area of the precentral motor cortex (Broca's area). The patient is not fluent but comprehends speech well, shows poor repetition, poor naming of recognized objects, evidences a scant, telegraphic speech, usually cannot write, and would be expected to have a right hemiparesis.

3. Transcortical aphasias: caused by a crescentic infarction between the watersheds of the middle and anterior cerebral artery seen in cerebral anoxia. The patient repeats well. In the motor variety, he is not fluent but comprehends speech. In the sensory variety, he is fluent but has no comprehension.

4. Wernicke's (receptive, sensory) aphasia: involvement of the posterior portion of the superior temporal gyrus. Patient is fluent, does not comprehend speech, cannot repeat, produces neologisms, is unaware of his disabilities or situation, and has poor reading and writing ability.

5. Conduction aphasia: due to a lesion involving the subcortical connections from the parietal to frontal lobe between interhemispheric cortex and basal nuclei. The patient is fluent, comprehends speech, repeats poorly (especially short words and phrases).

6. Amnesic aphasia: The patient has difficulty with nouns or prepositional parts of speech and names of objects. It is a common aphasic or communication deficit that can be seen with motor cortex, parietal cortex, and diffuse cortical lesions.

These are only the major or frequent varieties of communication disorder. Further discussions can be found in works cited in the Bibliography. The problem with this approach is that it can impede communication between those working with the patient, and inhibit an appreciation of the true nature of the patient's lesion because: (1) the terms are often loosely and inappropriately used without determining the exactness of applicability to the patient; (2) the terms are often defined differently by different examiners; (3) patients rarely seem to fit these syndromes. As has been mentioned above, each patient is unique in the wiring of the cortex and the nature of the lesion. Use of the terms may prevent important signs in the patient from being observed or appreciated. This is a problem with eponyms in general!

It would be best for the examiner to list the communication disorders he finds in the patient as accurately as possible and state his assumption as to where in the brain the problem is located.

Disorders of communication skill caused by associative cortex damage should be differentiated from several conditions with which they can be confused: dysarthria, due to brain stem or bilateral corticobulbar dysfunction; psychoses; and the organic brain syndrome.

1. The dysarthric patient can marshall all the proper words for communication in the proper order but has difficulty in enunciation, even to the point of unintelligibility. The patient with a communication disorder usually enunciates words well, although a word or its use may be inappropriate or pointless. The dysarthric patient has no defect in understanding communication from the examiner. Nevertheless, with certain patients, particularly those with poor fluency due to anterior associative cortex damage, the two conditions may be impossible to differentiate. In patients with bilateral brain disease, they often coexist. The examiner should be certain he is not dealing with an apraxia of the tongue or speech.

2. Psychoses may be suggested by the behavior of the patient with loss of communication skills. Those patients with poor fluency due to precentral lesions often seem mute and withdrawn and occasionally may rage or cry when unable to express themselves. However, they are acutely aware of their difficulty. Those

with increased fluency due to posteriorly located lesions may appear psychotic in that they may not understand verbal instructions and may babble volumes of speech simulating the tangential, neologistic speech of the schizophrenic. The most helpful differential point is that the psychotic patient never seems to be in the same world with the examiner. The patient with defective cortical communication, by contrast, usually shows eagerness to communicate by any modality, and will work constantly with the interested examiner despite all obstacles.

3. The confusion of the organic brain syndrome may simulate a communication disorder. However, the organic brain syndrome is characterized by reduced consciousness, blunted affect and depressed awareness, general disorientation, wavering contact with the examiner, and lack of awareness of inappropriate responses. In addition, a history of progressive personality change is suggestive of the organic brain syndrome. The structure of the patient's response is often helpful; the patient with the organic brain syndrome frequently gives irrelevant responses in terms of context, but the words and syntax are intact. The patient with a communication disorder, on the other hand, shows considerable difficulty with words, sounds, and syntax but is attempting relevant communication. The faulty words used by the patient with a communication disorder are often not as irrelevant as initially apparent, in that they frequently sound like the correct word, may begin with the same letter as the correct word, or in some way are in the same category as an aspect of the correct word.

9

THE POORLY RESPONSIVE PATIENT

Coma or progressive unconsciousness is a neurological emergency that may be the result of a large number of factors shown in the following list.

Some Causes of Coma

Concussion, contusion
Expanding intracerebral lesion
    Tumor
    Hematoma (subdural, epidural)
    Abscess
    Cerebral edema
Intracranial bleeding
    Ruptured congenital aneurysm
    Intracerebral hemorrhage
Anoxia
Toxic exposure
    Alcohol
    Carbon monoxide
    Barbiturates
    Bromides
    Other drug abuse
Vascular insufficiency or circulatory failure
    Shock (reflex, cardiogenic, septic)
    Hemorrhage
Metabolic derangement
    Diabetic coma
    Hypoglycemia
    Hepatic coma
    Water intoxication
    Hyponatremia
Postictal state
Encephalitis

These etiologies have in common a structural or functional effect on the ascending reticular activating system. Coma is life-threatening; a rapid efficient means of evaluating unconsciousness is mandatory. The following routine is suggested.

EXAMINATION OF THE POORLY RESPONSIVE PATIENT

History

All immediately available historical facts from any source (*e.g.*, police, observers, ambulance drivers) must be obtained:

Rapidity and nature of coma's onset (complaints of patient, appearance of patient, progression of activities that led to coma)
Alcohol use
Drug use
Prior seizures
Previous coronary or cerebrovascular disease
Trauma to the head
Hypertension
Unvented gas heater or other sources of inhalable poisons (*e.g.*, carbon monoxide, methane)
Known diabetes

If attempts at obtaining information in these areas are nonproductive, move on to other aspects of the problem.

Patency of airway and ventilatory ability

Color of skin (cyanosis, cherry red color)
Slack jaw obstructing the airway
Pooled secretions in the pharynx
Accessory respiratory muscle activity
Rate, depth, and pattern of respiration (intercostals, diaphragm, accessory muscles)

Circulatory status

Color of skin (pallor, cyanosis)
Blood pressure and pulse
Cardiac examination (electrocardiogram)
Evidences of hemorrhage (rigid abdomen, melena, hematuria, blood in vomitus)

Enough blood should be drawn for analysis in necessary laboratory tests:

Complete blood count
Hemoglobin
Hematocrit
Blood glucose
Blood urea nitrogen

Electrolytes
Toxins (sedatives, barbiturates, alcohol, tranquilizers, bromides)
Carboxyhemoglobin

Intravenous infusion should be started so that if subsequent events indicate need for blood, electrolytes, or medication, they can be added. Blood for glucose determination should be drawn before glucose is given.

Trauma

The patient should be examined for evidence of trauma to the head and body, the head should be palpated, and ears and nose examined carefully for evidence of blood or cerebrospinal fluid. The possibility of a spinal fracture must be ruled out before the head is manipulated.

Infection

Temperature
Rash
Nuchal rigidity (meningeal signs may be due to subarachoid hemorrhage)

Intracranial pressure

Papilledema
Preretinal hemorrhage
Echoencephalogram shift
Pupillary dilation or unresponsiveness

Pupils should not be dilated since the loss of pupillary reflex and dilation of the pupil are cardinal, and often the only signs of impending brain stem compression.

Hypoglycemia

The possibility of hypoglycemia should be ruled out with 50 cc. of intravenous 50% glucose solution. This cannot hurt the patient, but undetected hypoglycemia can cause progressively irreversible cerebral damage. Hypoglycemia can produce a variety of neurological deficits. Blood for determination of glucose levels must be drawn before glucose solution is administered.

Diabetes

The possibility of diabetes should be ruled out, if possible, by evaluation of history, urine, and blood.

General physical assessment

Examination for petechiae, ecchymoses, marks of suicide attempt, needle punctures, and laceration of the tongue caused by seizures.
Rectal examination for blood or bloody stool
Possible laboratory examination of all vomitus, feces, and urine.

Confirmatory Tests

If the workup at this point has indicated a nonneurological cause for coma (*e.g.*, diabetes, cardiac arrest, anoxia, suicide attempt, shock, myocardial infarction), the appropriate confirmatory tests should be undertaken (*e.g.*, blood studies, electrocardiogram) and therapy given.

Neurological Examination

Level of Consciousness Level of consciousness must be documented carefully to determine whether the patient is worsening or improving. The following somewhat arbitrary stages help to characterize the findings in patients without focal neurological signs, from alertness to deep coma:

1. Fully alert
2. Rousable to appropriate motor or verbal responses; follows commands
   Oriented
   Spontaneous speech (appropriate?, understandable?)
   Illusions, delusions, hallucinations
   Reduced awareness of environment
   Restlesness
3. Spontaneous movement
   Responsive to many stimuli, external and internal
   Occasionally combative
   Repeated verbal stimuli may produce appropriate answers
   Variable sphincter control
4. Response to pain that is "organized" or "psychologically understable" (*i.e.*, turning face or moving limb away from stimulus)
   Persistant stimuli (*e.g.*, shake, yell) may produce verbal mumblings
   Incontinence of urine and feces
   Reflexes intact
   No speech
5. Response to severe pain with vague movements or decerebrate posture (may also have pupillary, deep tendon reflexes, plantar responses, and fluctuating vital signs)
6. No pain response
   No reflexes
   No pupillary responses
   Fluctuating vital signs

AKINETIC MUTISM

With severe bilateral frontal or subfrontal lesions, the patient may become extremely withdrawn, akinetic, and mute, and may often stare blankly ahead showing little response to environment or any stimulation. The patient will respond to constant urging, and will chew and swallow if fed. Occasional vocalizations will occur.

VIGILANT COMA ("Locked in" Syndrome)

With diencephalic lesions, as seen in patients with anoxia or high brain-stem lesions ventrally placed, the patient is "locked in" or totally incapable of speech or movement due to bilateral corticobulbar and corticospinal involvement. Yet, despite "comatose" appearance and behavior, they are usually conscious and aware of their surroundings. The examiner can suspect this state by the characteristic eyes-open appearance of these patients. They may be unblinking (reptilian stare). The examiner has the feeling that, by his appearance, the patient is apt to speak at any time, but he never does. Further documentation can be made if the patient can close/open the eyes or move the eyes on command. One patient was recognized as being in vigilant coma by tearing when her name was mentioned. These patients often show decerebrate phenomena. The recognition and differentiation of this condition is crucial, as these patients are conscious. Personnel working and talking at the bedside must keep this in mind.

Optic Nerve Funduscopic examination is essential in all patients to look for:

Papilledema, hemorrhage, exudates
Visual field by threat

Oculomotor Nerves

Pupillary size and responses
Ptosis
Spontaneous movements of eyes: conjugate, dysconjugate, oriented, roving
Oculocephalic responses on head turning. (Eyes should deviate to side away from direction in which the examiner rotates the head.)
Caloric response to ice water douched into the ear (oculovestibular response). (Be sure the tympanic membrane is intact. Lack of any response may be seen in deep coma. Bizarre or exaggerated eye responses indicate brain stem involvement, especially if bilateral.)

Trigeminal Nerve

Corneal reflex
Jaw reflex
Jaw tone

Facial Nerve

Facial symmetry
Assymetrical blowing of the lips
Grimace on painful stimuli (bilaterally)
Orbicularis oculi reflexes

Auditory Nerve Stethoscope in patient's ears; blinking when vibrating tuning fork is applied to diaphragm

Glossopharyngeal and Vagus Nerves

Gag reflex bilaterally
Swallowing reflex

Spontaneous Involuntary Motor Movements

Postures; flexion, extension (limbs, neck, trunk)
Myoclonus
Spasms
Seizures, focal or general

Decerebrate response (unilateral or bilateral—may be aggravated by manipulation or painful stimuli.)
Tetany
Fasciculations

Motor Impairment

Voluntary movements on command
Movement on painful stimuli
Extremity tonus (spasticity, rigidity, hypertonicity, or flaccidity)
Neck-turning reflexes (effect of head-turning on posture and tonus of limbs)
Attempted guarding when arm is dropped toward the face
Atrophy, fasciculation
Leg drop (muscular control of fall)

Respiratory Pattern

Rate, depth
Regular, periodic, ataxic

Reflexes

Deep tendon
Superficial abdominal
Plantar responses
Snout, palmomental, glabellar, grasp, etc.

Sensation
Reaction to stimuli

Meningeal Signs
Neural rigidity

Bruit in head

Palpation of great vessels
Auscultation of great vessels

BRAIN STEM DYSFUNCTION WITH SUPRATENTORIAL MASS LESIONS OR INCREASED INTRACRANIAL PRESSURE

All examiners of comatose patients should be aware of the signs and symptoms of impending brain stem failure caused by increased supratentorial intracranial pressure of any cause transmitted down the posterior fossa. This dysfunction travels in a caudad direction ending in death with medullary failure. Plum advocates the following observations to monitor the patient's status in this situation:*

Respiration
Pupillary size and light response
Pupillary response to neck pinch ipsilaterally (ciliospinal reflex)
Oculocephalic reflex on head turning
Gaze response to ice water calorics

*McNealy, D. S., and Plum, F.: "Brainstem dysfunction with supratenorial mass lesions." Arch. Neurol., 7:10-32, 1962. (also see Bibliography)

Response to supraorbital nerve pressure
Reflexes and muscle tone

He characterized the following findings for various anatomic levels of brain stem dysfunction.

Early Diencephalic

Normal or Cheyne-Strokes respirations
Small pupils bilaterally with light response
Present ciliospinal refelx
Present oculocephalics (may be sluggish)
Ipsilateral gaze to ice water caloric with loss of quick component in nystagmus
Appropriate pain response (e.g., avoidance, resistance)
Bilateral extensor plantars and gegenhalten in extremities

Late Diencephalic (Only changes from above noted)

Cheyne-Strokes respiration
Small pupils bilaterally with light response
Present ciliospinal reflex
Present oculocephalics, but more pronounced
Present caloric response, but more pronounced
Decorticate rigidity (arms flexed, legs extended)

Midbrain-Upper Pons

Regular hyperventilation
Midposition, irregular pupils, no response
No response to ciliospinal reflex
Impaired oculocephalics
Impaired or dysconjugate caloric response
Lack of pain response

The examiner should be aware also of signs of uncal herniation caused by supratentorial pressure. The uncal tip of the temporal lobe may pass over the edge of the tentorium in the tentorial notch and compress the third nerve, causing first an intraocular ophthalmoplegia noted as a progressively dilating and unresponsive ipsilateral pupil. This is superimposed by extraocular ophthalmoplegia as the ipsilateral eye fails to adduct on oculocephalic and caloric testing. The temporal herniation then compresses the midbrain and causes the findings mentioned above. With catastrophic increases in pressure as seen in intraventricular hemorrhage, the sequence of events described may not be followed or move very rapidly. The life-threatening nature of these findings makes it imperative that the examiner be well versed in examination.

Downward deviated eyes with small nonreacting pupils are seen with bilateral thalamic hemorrhages. Tonically deviated eyes are seen with acute contralateral cerebral lesions. Pinpoint pupils, especially associated with skew deviation of the eyes, suggest a pontine lesion. Midbrain lesions are associated with fixed, midposition pupils and again skew deviation of the eyes may be seen.

In metabolic or toxic comas, the eyes may rove from side to side. The oculocephalic and oculovestibular responses may be intact or totally absent. In the latter situation, unlike space-occupying lesions, pupil reaction may still be seen.

Bizarre oculovestibular or oculocephalic responses may be seen with a variety of brain stem lesions, tonic deviation of the eyes, monocular or asymmetric deviation, or no response unilaterally or bilaterally. Acute cerebellar lesions may show deviated, skew, or normal eye responses, and the pupils can range from normal to pinpoint.

These ocular findings can serve as guidelines but are not invariable, and, as always, the entire picture the patient presents has to be put together.

10

REPORTING THE NEUROLOGICAL EXAMINATION

THE NORMAL EXAMINATION

This section is included to suggest the minimum neurological assessment when no positive signs are found. It will also help the examiner decide on the minimum examination necessary to survey or scan for other possible neurological deficits after he has concentrated on the patient's principle problem. Even in the general physical assessment of the patient, this could be considered a guide to the minimum examination of the nervous system. If an abnormality is discovered on scanning or routine examination, the examiner must expand his investigation of that area utilizing the techniques described previously. For example, if a ticking watch was not heard equally on both sides, then the examiner would have to proceed with the Rinne and Weber examinations. If a communication disorder is suggested, or diplopia is evidenced, then considerable work lies ahead for the examiner.

The recorded history should represent an accurate translation and abstraction of the patient's illness mindful of all the concerns set forth earlier about temporal profile, earliest onset of symptoms, family history, review of all possible neurological symptoms, and an accurate dissection of the patient's own use of symptoms.

The suggested report for a negative examination is as follows:

The patient is alert, cooperative, intelligent and well oriented without evidence of a communication disorder. Body posture and activity do not seem unusual.

Cranial Nerves

I Smell is intact ____ being identified on the right and ____ on the left.
II The patient reads small print bilaterally. Visual fields are intact to confrontation. Funduscopic: the disc is pinkish-yellow, the margins are sharp, and there is a moderate amount of physiological cupping bilaterally. The vessels and retinae seem unremarkable.

III, IV, VI The pupils are round, equal and react quickly and equally to light and convergence. Extraocular movements are full. The patient does not complain of diplopia, and shows no evidence of dysconjugate gaze.

     V The jaw does not deviate. Sensation is intact and corneal reflex is active bilaterally. Jaw jerk is 1+.

   VII There is no weakness of the facial muscles on voluntary or reflex movement.

  VIII Watch heard well bilaterally.

  IX, X The palate rises equally bilaterally. There is no difficulty in swallowing or speaking. Gag reflex is active bilaterally. Pharyngeal sensation intact bilaterally.

    XI Sternomastoid and trapezius muscles are strong and equal bilaterally.

   XII The tongue protrudes in the midline, with no atrophy or fasciculations. No evidence of dysarthria or speech impairment.

Meningeal Signs

The neck is supple. No pain or restriction of straight leg raising.

Motor Systems

No abnormality is noted. Strength, coordination and muscle tone are good throughout. No fasciculations or atrophy are seen. There are no cerebellar or extrapyramidal signs.

Sensory Systems

Light touch, position sense, pin, vibration sense, stereognosis, and the Romberg test are all negative.

Reflexes

Deep tendon reflexes are active and equal throughout without evidence of clonus. Plantar response are flexor bilaterally, and the superficial abdominal reflexes are intact. No pathological reflexes are seen.

Gait and Station

Gait, station, and posture are unremarkable; no skeletal abnormalities are noted.

No abnormalities are found on examination of palpable arteries and nerves. No bruits are heard over the head and neck.

11

THE NEUROLOGIST'S CLINICAL REASONING PROCESS
(Putting It All Together)

When the neurologist first encounters a patient with a suspected neurological problem, he immediately assembles a number of perceived cues into an initial concept of the patient's problem. These cues are taken from the patient (appearance, complaints, comments, dress, manner, movements) and accompanying notes or laboratory data. For the experienced clinician, this perception of cues and the synthesis into an initial concept is automatic and largely unconscious. Cue perception is not a passive process, since important cues may not call attention to themselves; they have to be sought. The neurologist's past experiences with patients, and his knowledge of neurological diseases, cause him to look for certain cues with a patient's particular complaint or problem. Although the clinician's initial concept of the problem is often the same as the patient's initial complaint, it can be quite different if he perceives other cues (*e.g.*, a dysarthric voice, a slight facial weakness, an anxious appearance, confused behavior). The student, who may not have prior experiences with patients or a depth of knowledge to draw from, needs to consciously and methodically search the patient and the patient's environment for important cues to assemble into his initial concept of the patient's problem.

The initial concept serves as a trigger for the experienced examiner's long-term memory banks, causing a number of hypotheses that could explain his initial concept of the patient's problem to pop into his mind. These multiple hypotheses can be vague, such as "something wrong in the left hemisphere," or a focused and specific hypothesis such as "myotonia dystrophica." It is characteristic of the neurologist to initially entertain a number of hypotheses concerning anatomical localization. For example, if his initial concept in an emergency room situation is "a young girl with an acute paralysis of both legs," the multiple hypotheses that flash in his head might be: (1) spinal cord lesion; (2) Guillain-Barré syndrome; (3) periodic paralysis; (4) hysterical paralysis, (5) multiple sclerosis. Of course these would vary from neurologist to neurologist because of varying prior personal experiences with such a problem. These multiple hypotheses serve as possible patterns or templates that may ultimately fit the patient's problem depending upon further information that will be obtained from history, examination, and subsequent tests. Each hypothesis represents a possible end point for the evaluation of the patient. As a group, they serve as a guide for the next questions the neurologist is going to ask the patient or for the aspects of neurological examination he will perform.

This formation of multiple hypotheses is the creative step in the evaluation of the patient, where pattern recognition, "divergent thinking," or "brainstorming" can play an important role. It is important for the student to develop an ability to hypothesize widely from his initial concept of the patient. He should search his long-term memory banks for relevant associations or ideas from past experience and knowledge to serve as hypotheses. In this way, he will strengthen his ability to create a sufficient number of hypotheses so that he can select the best four or five with which to work. Multiple hypotheses make the problem-solving process efficient and accurate. To help with this creative process, the student should review possible anatomical locations for his initial concept of the problem, such as cortex, hemisphere, brainstem, cerebellum, spinal cord, root, peripheral nerve, myoneural junction, muscle, right or left or bilateral locations, and focal or multifocal or diffuse lesions.

In the case of a young girl with paralysis in the legs, the student may consider spinal cord, multiple lumbosacral roots, peripheral nerves, myoneural junction, or muscle, until a few initial questions or examination narrow down the possibilities. Once he has done this, the student should then review a similar list of possible etiologies for neurological disease, such as congenital, genetic, neoplastic, cardiovascular, metabolic, psychiatric or psychological, traumatic, toxic, demyelination, infectious, degenerative or unknown, periodic or idiopathic (seizures, migraine, narcolepsy), and immunologic.

Again, with the young paraplegic girl, traumatic, psychiatric, infectious, demyelination, or metabolic causes might be considered by the student. As the student builds experience and knowledge, and exercises his hypothesis generation skill, he will begin to have useful, relevant multiple hypotheses jump into his mind as a guide for his evaluation of the patient. Parenthetically, the student must be certain that his future experiences with patients, and the information gained by study, are incorporated into his understanding of the various anatomical and etiological entities he may use as hypotheses to strengthen the organization of his memory.

The next step taken by the clinician, armed with his initial concept of the problem and multiple hypotheses as a guide, is to employ an inquiry strategy. This requires a change in thinking from a creative, horizontal, or free-associative approach to a convergent, vertical, analytical, or deductive approach. The task at this stage is to employ, from the thousands of questions that could be asked or items of neurological examination that could be performed, those inquiries that will most rapidly and accurately determine whether or not the patient's problem matches any of his multiple hypotheses. The experienced clinician has developed a variety of almost automatic strategies to quickly clarify the nature of a variety of problems.

With the paraplegic girl, he might inquire about sensory loss in the legs. If present, this would strengthen the hypothesis of spinal cord or root disease and eliminate periodic paralysis, myasthenia, or myopathy. He might inquire about bladder or bowel symptoms to strengthen the spinal cord hypothesis and weaken the hypothesis of root disease such as Guillain-Barré. To develop this skill, the student must consider the evidence that would shape the patient's problem to the patterns suggested by his hypotheses. Inquiry about the exact nature of the symptoms, the temporal profile of the symptoms, and other associated symptoms assist in this process. In this inquiry, the examiner will receive a growing body of information in response to his questions and examinations, much of which will need to be retained. The information that is relevant to his hypotheses, and contributes to clarifying the patient's particular problem pattern, is added to his initial concept. The initial concept, as a consequence, continues to grow in the mind or working memory alongside his hypotheses and becomes the patient's problem pattern. The clinician must shape the unique picture the patient presents by his inquiry strategy in a manner that allows him to see if it fits any of his hypotheses. If, in this process, he confirms one of his more general hypotheses, the clinician replaces that hypothesis with a new group of more specific multiple hypotheses to see how finely he can evaluate or diagnose the patient's problem. For example, if the girl describes urinary urgency followed by retention, sensory loss to the waist, and evidences bilateral extensor plantars, the general hypothesis of spinal cord lesion would seem confirmed. At this point, new hypotheses would pop into the clinician's head, such as spinal cord tumor (intramedullary, extramedullary, primary, secondary), transverse myelitis, multiple sclerosis, intramedullary hemorrhage (arteriovenous malformation, syringomyelia), and a new inquiry strategy begins.

On many occasions, the examiner may hit a blind alley in his inquiry and might not be able to confirm or deny his hypotheses, or might find that he can deny all his hypotheses. At this point, the clinician scans for new information that could provide new cues that may reshape the patient's problem pattern and produce new hypotheses. He usually does this by reviewing the patient's story and by making routine inquiries about other possible neurological symptoms, symptoms of other body system dysfunctions (*e.g.,* cardiovascular, gastrointestinal, renal), past history, family history, and social history. A new cue produces new hypotheses and sets the inquiry or search process into action again. Alternatively, the clinician might reconsider some of the more remote hypotheses he discarded earlier in his need to work with a handful of the more likely, more important, or more treatable hypotheses.

The neurological examination is usually carried out after a period of initial interview. However, in some situations, it is linked with the history to make the inquiry strategy more efficient. In the young paraplegic, the early finding of loss of sensation to the waist on pin-prick and extensor plantar responses bilaterally would eliminate the need, in the emergency room, for the inevitably lengthy inquiry about psychological factors to adequately consider a hysterical paralysis. Nevertheless, when performed after the interview, the neurological examination is usually focused to confirm the one or two hypotheses entertained by the clinician at the end of his interview. The experienced neurologist knows exactly what he is going to look for on the examination and what he expects to find. With the paraplegic girl, he probably would (1) confirm the paralysis and determine its upper level; (2) examine reflexes and muscle tone to establish whether the paralysis is due to upper or lower motor neuron involvement; (3) establish the sensory modalities affected and their pattern, particularly seeking saddle sparing to confirm an intermedullary lesion; (4) palpate the abdomen for a distended bladder; and (5) survey the cranial nerves.

Throughout this inquiry process, the clinician will usually establish the most probable hypothesis or hypotheses for his patient's problem as his diagnostic impression and decide on a subsequent course of tests and treatments. Before he concludes, he will perform a routine scan, similar to that mentioned to find new hypotheses, to be certain he has not missed any evidence that could suggest further problems, or change his decision. The clinician does this to gain confidence in his diagnostic decision. The extent of this routine inquiry or scanning depends on the time available, the urgency of the problem, the complexity of the problem, the clinician's security in his diagnostic decisions, and his natural compulsiveness. Some clinicians may begin with such routine inquiry to establish rapport with the patient. It's all a matter of style. Once he has finished the evaluation, the same inquiry strategy is employed to choose appropriate tests and diagnostic procedures.

The cyclic process continues until a decision is made concerning diagnosis and treatment. The process is truncated to meet emergency situations requiring very efficient and effective inquiry actions, and often requiring intervention or treatment of symptoms or signs before anything resembling a diagnosis can be made. In complex, chronic problems the process may extend over many examination sessions, and the inquiry process might involve numerous diagnostic tests, therapeutic trials, consultations, and management plans. Nevertheless, in all instances the basic process is the same. The experienced clinician does not make many precise diagnoses prior to more definitive tests. This is why the term "diagnosis" should be avoided. It is better to use terms such as "impression," "problem formulation," or, most likely, "hypothesis." Making a precise diagnosis when it is not warranted by the available data is a mistake that can actually inhibit effective evaluation.

In summary, the previous chapters have provided the techniques necessary for gathering data from the patient, and have provided some information on how the data can be analyzed in terms of lesion localization. This last chapter has discussed the overall problem-solving approach of the neurologist to put these techniques into perspective. These techniques should be employed as appropriate in the clinician's inquiry strategy. His inquiry strategy is problem oriented; the questions and examinations are martialed in a sequence appropriate to uncovering the data needed to evoke multiple hypotheses in the examiner's mind. There is no such thing as a routine neurological examination. The technique of the neurological examination should serve the examiner in his inquiry, and not be imposed upon the patient as a ritual. If the examiner does not know what he should be looking for, he probably won't find it. The only routine that exists is the scanning necessary to be certain other cues have not been overlooked.

To become proficient in the neurological examination, the student must seek more and more experience with patients. With each patient's problem he should:

1. Look for initial cues.
2. Assemble them into an *initial concept* of the problem.
3. Generate *multiple hypotheses* that may explain the cause or nature of the problem (with initial emphasis on anatomical hypotheses).
4. Employ an *inquiry strategy* aimed at providing information about the patient's problem that will determine its fit to the hypotheses generated.

5. Incorporate the information acquired into an evolving *problem pattern* that can be compared to the *multiple hypotheses*.
6. If there is no fit, or the hypotheses prove unlikely, scan for more data to suggest new hypotheses.
7. Continue these activities until confident of the correct hypothesis, or hypotheses, and then decide on the appropriate further *inquiry strategy* with tests and diagnostic procedures (mindful of cost, risk, and payoff diagnostically).
8. When the diagnosis or patient's problem has been discovered, the student should review this experience in terms of what new understanding he may have achieved about neural form and function, and the adequacy/inadequacy of the hypotheses he employed.

BIBLIOGRAPHY

Some Sources of Detailed Information in Special Areas
of the Neurological Examination

Baloh, R. W., and Honrubia, V.: Clinical Neurophysiology of the Vestibular System. Philadelphia, F. A. Davis, 1979.
Geschwind, N.: Aphasia, current concepts. N. Engl. J. Med., 284:654, 1971.
Glaser, J. S.: Neurophthalmology. Hagerstown, Harper & Row, 1978.
Plum, F., and Posner, J. B.: Diagnosis of Stupor and Coma. ed. 2. Philadelphia, F. A. Davis, 1972.
Strub, R. L., and Black, F. W.: The Mental Status Examination in Neurology. Philadelphia, F. A. Davis, 1977.

Sources of Problem Solving or Clinical Reasoning
for the Neurologist

Barrows, H. S., and Bennett, K.: Experimental studies on the diagnostic (problem solving) skill of the neurologist. Arch. Neurol., 26:273, 1972.
Barrows, H. S., Neufeld, V. R., Feightner, J. W., and Norman, G. R.: Analysis of the Clinical Methods of Medical Students and Physicians. Hamilton, McMaster University, 1978.
Elstein, A. S., Shulman, L. S., and Sprafka, S. A.: An Analysis of Clinical Reasoning. Cambridge, Harvard University Press, 1978.
Kleinmuntz, B.: The processing of clinical information by man and machine. In B. Kleinmuntz (Ed.). Formal Representation of Human Judgment. New York, John Wiley, 1968. Pittsburgh, Carnegie Mellon University, 1968.

INDEX

Numerals in *italics* indicate a figure.

153